Communication
in the
Nursing Context
Third Edition

Communication
in the
Nursing Context
Third Edition

Jean C. Bradley, R.N., Ph.D.
Interim Assistant Dean, Regional Nursing Program
Associate Professor of Medical–Surgical Nursing
College of Nursing
University of Illinois
Peoria, Illinois

Mark A. Edinberg, Ph.D.
Director, Center for the Study of Aging
Professor of Gerontology
College of Health and Human Services
University of Bridgeport
Bridgeport, Connecticut

APPLETON & LANGE
Norwalk, Connecticut/San Mateo, California

0-8385-1327-1

Prentice Hall International (UK) Limited, *London*
Prentice-Hall of Australia, Pty. Limited, *Sydney*
Prentice-Hall Canada, Inc., *Toronto*
Prentice-Hall Hispanoamericana, S. A., *Mexico*
Prentice-Hall of India Private Limited, *New Delhi*
Prentice-Hall of Japan, Inc., *Tokyo*
Simon & Schuster Asia Pte. Ltd., *Singapore*
Editora Prentice Hall do Brasil Ltda., *Rio de Janeiro*
Prentice Hall, *Englewood Cliffs, New Jersey*

Library of Congress Cataloging-in-Publication Data

Bradley, Jean C., 1927–
　　Communication in the nursing context / Jean C. Bradley, Mark A. Edinberg. — 3rd ed.
　　　　p.　cm.
　　Includes bibliographical references.
　　ISBN 0-8385-1327-1
　　1. Communication in nursing.　2. Communication—nurses' instruction.　I. Edinberg, Mark A., 1947–　.　II. Title.
　　[DNLM:　WY　87　B811c]
　　RT23.B7　　　1990
　　302.2'024613—dc20
　　DNLM/DLC
　　for Library of Congress　　　　　　　　　　　　　　　　89-18424
　　　　　　　　　　　　　　　　　　　　　　　　　　　　　　CIP

Acquisitions Editor: Marion Kalstein-Welch
Production Editor: Sandra K. Huggard
Designer: Michael J. Kelly

PRINTED IN THE UNITED STATES OF AMERICA

Contents

Preface

Over a decade has passed since we began the initial work on the first edition of this communication text. In retrospect, we are amazed by the changes that have occurred, not only in nursing, but in the total health care delivery system. In 1979, few persons, if any, had heard of Acquired Immune Deficiency Syndrome (AIDS) or Diagnostic Related Groups (DRGs). Today, clients are suffering new disease entities and leaving the hospital in shorter periods of time. For nurses to successfully demonstrate their skills with advanced technology and thus the ability to care for clients, they must communicate with other nurses, clients and their families, and with other health professionals.

The text, for its primary purpose, relates theoretical communication concepts to clinical nursing problems. The text retains certain essential characteristics from previous editions, including a strong theoretical and practice orientation. In addition, every exercise in the text is directly related to nursing process issues. The content, we believe, is relevant to all nurses—beginning and advanced students as well as graduate nurses on different levels.

The text divides into four major sections. The **first section** introduces communication content organized around King's nursing theory. Satir's communication framework is applied to the nursing context; a neurolinguistic approach is introduced through the use of channels, and interviewing skills are described.

The **second section** addresses communication between nurses and others in a variety of role relationships, including different applicable techniques (e.g., assertion).

The **third section** addresses communication in different settings: hospital, ambulatory, or home care settings. This section discusses different group interactions, including the families of patients.

The **fourth section** and last, includes several areas related to communication that are new to this third edition, for instance: home-based communication, AIDS patients, substance abuse patients, abused children, elderly, cultural and ethnic groups, chemically dependent clients, and health promotion.

The text's content is highlighted with exercises and discussion topics. The exercises can be used by the instructor to provide students learning opportunities and practice in communication skills. Advanced students or graduate nurses may choose not to participate directly; however, we believe that reading the content of the exercise will contribute to their learning experiences.

The organization of the text progresses from basic to more complex. Each chapter lists behavioral objectives enabling students and instructors an evaluation of the material learned. Many of the references have been updated. We attempted throughout the text to eliminate bias when dealing with sex, ethnicity, or health occupations. For example, we portray a male nurse and a female physician in several vignettes.

We hope we have helped nurses deal more effectively with communication breakdowns that occur in different settings and in role relationships with different clients. As we approach the 21st century, we believe that changes will be ever more rapid and that communication, a key ingredient in the nursing process, will continue as a vital component for transmitting and understanding advanced technology.

We would like to thank our editor, Marion Kalstein-Welch, for her guidance throughout the preparation of this edition, and our production editor, Sandra K. Huggard. We also want to thank our families—Barbara, Joel, and Daniel Edinberg and Arthur and K.C. Bradley—who not only were tolerant of our time spent on the revision, but also helped with effective listening skills as we involved them in the process. Finally, we thank Linnet Graze, an administrative secretary at the University of Illinois, who always provided encouragement and assistance when needed.

Jean C. Bradley, R.N., Ph.D.
Mark A. Edinberg, Ph.D.

	# Communication Competencies
Section I	

The first section of this book presents communication competencies and the relationship of these competencies to the conceptual framework of the nursing process. Examining the way in which the nurse and client become actively involved in each of the four phases of the nursing process—*assessment, plan, implementation,* and *evaluation*—we see that communication is the common thread tying these phases together. To communicate is to understand both verbal and nonverbal messages; it is the ability to share experiences with another and to set mutually chosen goals with the client. Communication implies not only understanding the unique needs of each client, but interacting with other health care professionals as well.

The purpose of Section I is to provide a foundation of knowledge upon which effective communication skills can then be developed. Chapters 1 through 3 provide the student with a fundamental knowledge of individual dynamics in the communication process. Chapter 4 is designed to give the student a beginning comprehension of the techniques for interviewing. And Chapter 5 presents information designed to help students gain an increase in their capacity for self-understanding and for their "professional use of self."

1 Communication and Nursing Models

BEHAVIORAL OBJECTIVES

By reading this chapter and participating in the exercises, students will be able to:

1. Describe the five elements of a generic communication model
2. Demonstrate an understanding of the basic principles of communication (as proposed by Watzlawick et al., 1967)
3. Explain the differences between one-way and two-way communication
4. Describe the three interacting systems in King's nursing theory
5. Describe the relationship of the steps in the nursing process to communication
6. Identify three clusters of nursing actions and relate them to the nursing process
7. Explain the concept of "degrees of visibility" in relation to nursing actions

A nurse working on a surgical unit in a hospital is assigned the following client:

> Mary Cole, a 32-year-old mother of two children, had a mastectomy 2 days ago. She has had a rapid physical recovery, and as the nurse assists her to sit up on the side of the bed prior to ambulation, Mary states, "I'm really worried about what caused this illness. I don't think it was the smoking. Anyway, I don't intend to stop that now. What do you think?"

What should the nurse say or do in this situation? It is important to have several questions answered before venturing a response to what is obviously not a simple question. The nurse who is taking care of Mary would want to know how much she has been told about her condition by others, including her physician. He or she would also want to know Mary's reactions to her diagnosis and operation to date and what physical progress she has been making in relation to her operation. He or she might even want to know what Mary's disposition has been for the last 24 hours.

Even with all that information, the nurse would still have many options for responding. Several that seem appropriate include:

- Taking her hand, sitting next to her and asking, "What is your concern?"
- Asking, "What would you like to know about smoking?"
- Pulling up a chair and waiting for her to continue.

Are there any other responses that seem appropriate and fitting? There are also several responses that do *not* seem appropriate:

- Walking away and pretending one doesn't hear her.
- Saying, "You look so healthy! Don't worry!"
- Saying, "Oh, you'll have to ask the doctor that," and moving away.

Are there others that would be inappropriate?

Nurses meet many Marys and find themselves in many situations where the "right" response is not automatically obvious. They need more information than is available; they will have to make educated guesses about what is meant and then "instantaneously" make a response to the situation.

As soon as the nurse makes a response, Mary, or anyone else will say or do something that requires another response from the nurse. This series of "situations" and "responses" can be called a communication sequence. Each response depends on the situation that preceded it. Furthermore, the nurse's response becomes the situation or "stimulus" to which Mary will respond. Any communication can be thought of as "interactive," that is, each piece of information is partly affected by the previous communication. So what the nurse says or does depends on what Mary said, as well as the communication skills and knowledge utilized in the particular situation.

After the nurse has figured out *what* to say, *how* might it be said? What tone of voice should be used? What specific words would be best? How would the nurse position arms, stand, or sit? How would he or she speak, or what facial expression would he or she use? Do nurses think about any of these questions or do they respond automatically?

Needless to say, if nurses went through the above list of questions and figured out answers to each of them before a response was made, it would take 3 to 5 minutes before they could say anything to Mary, who would, by that time, be thinking that something was wrong with the nurse! Nursing responses should be "automatic" *and* appropriate for the particular client. While the dissection of communication that is made in this book may tend to overanalyze the pieces, learnings ultimately have to become so integrated that the message sent will automatically reflect a nurse's knowledge of body language, communication channels, communication skills, communication styles, and role relationships. The student's responsibility as a learner is to try out the pieces and exercises presented in this book so that effective communication skills become part of his or her nursing repertoire.

How effectively nurses communicate with others is certainly one of the most, if not *the* most, important components of nursing practice. When we consider how often communication skills are utilized in a practicing profession such as nursing, we realize that nursing *is* communicating in the fullest sense—seeing, listening, and feeling.

In the course of this book some theoretical concepts, ideas, and specific strategies will be presented in order to make students more effective as nurse communicators. While the theoretical materials are important for thinking, the skills and exercises are perhaps even more important for clinical experience. Good communication requires practice as well as the development of several styles or types of responses so that one will be able to respond appropriately to what is seen, felt, and heard in all nursing experiences.

COMMUNICATION MODELS

Researchers and authors have broken up the communication sequence into smaller parts; these are often called elements or components. At other times, the pieces are more or less observations about aspects of communication. There is not necessarily one "correct" way to analyze communication, but each view can add its own understanding and, hopefully, expand our thinking and awareness about communication and nursing. Also, communication becomes more complicated the more it is examined. Consider the basic communication model in Figure 1–1, which consists of essential questions that can be asked about a communication process; who says *what*, to *whom*, in what *channel* with what *effect* (Laswell, 1948). The model also highlights five essential components of communication: source, message, channel, receiver, and feedback.

Who? The Sender. The individual who generates or sends the message is also referred to as the "source-encoder." The source is an idea, event, or situation. Encoding involves the selection of specific signs or symbols (codes) used in transmitting the message, such as the use of language.

For example, when the nurse asks the client, "Do you have pain?", the nurse is the sender. The idea that the client has pain is the source, and the use of language as well as placing a hand on the client's shoulder constitute encoding.

Communicates? The Message. The message consists of stimuli (verbal and nonverbal) that are generated by the source and responded to (or not responded to) by the receiver. Messages consist of words spoken (content) and nonverbal cues, for example, gestures, posture, tone of voice.

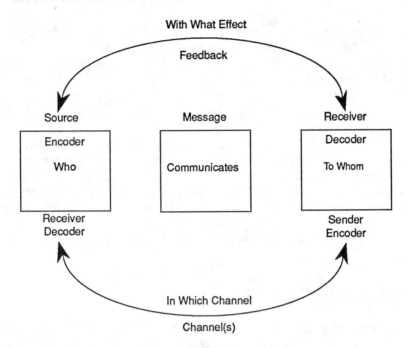

Figure 1–1. Communication Model.

In Which Channel? The Channel. The channel refers to the medium through which the message is transmitted. The three primary channels, which will be covered in Chapter 2, are visual (seeing), auditory (hearing), and kinesthetic (feeling).

To Whom? The Receiver. The individual who receives the message is also referred to as the "decoder." The receiver perceives what the sender intended (through the sensations of seeing, hearing, and feeling) and then analyzes the information (through interpretation of what is thought to be seen, heard, or felt). When we use language, our primary concern is with interpretation of the message. Since communication involves at least two people who are sending and receiving messages, each communicator in the process can be thought of as *both* a sender and receiver.

For example, the client (receiver) responds to the nurse's (sender) question, "Do you have pain?" by saying, "Yes, I feel terrible." The client thus becomes the sender and the nurse the receiver of the message.

With What Effect? Feedback. Feedback constitutes the information the sender receives about the receiver's reaction to the message that has been generated. Feedback is effective when the two communicators are sensitive to each other's message and modify their behavior accordingly. Changes in the sender's behavior that are reactions to the feedback that has been received are part of the total feedback process. In our example, the nurse receives the feedback and administers a pain medication.

One-Way and Two-Way Communication

Although almost all communication is interactive and dependent on the sender and receiver responses, people can act *as if* there is no feedback or response to whatever they are communicating. Thus, the flow of information is in one direction. This kind of communication is called "one-way."

One-way communication is quick, uncomplicated, and easy for the communicator to accomplish. In the health professions, people find themselves using one-way communication often and in a variety of settings: written memos, announcements over the public address system, physicians' and nurses' orders, nurses' end of shift report, nurses' procedure manual, and even in client education. Again, this method is quick, easy, and gives control to the communicator.

Often, clients with ongoing medical problems will need to monitor their own physical changes or take medication as part of a treatment plan. One of the most difficult issues in health care today is compliance in these areas. If the client education on self-monitoring, medication, or expected progress of the illness is given in a one-way fashion, nurses will not *really* know how much clients understand. A client may say "yes" when asked if he or she understood something only to find out the next day he or she did not understand it to the point of being able to remember it. Also, clients are likely to view nurses as evaluators who judge whether they are complying with their health regimens. Thus, a client may choose to wait until the next appointment (one-way), rather than providing feedback by calling in and reporting to the nurse when an untoward reaction occurs (two-way).

The alternative to one-way communication is two-way communication, in which the "recipient" becomes actively involved in the communication process, giving responses immediately to the message sender, who in turn can modify the next message based on the other's response (or "feedback"). The two-way process may be slower than one-way, it requires listening and flexibility on the part of the message sender, and it may be difficult to accomplish. A comparison of one-way and two-way communication is shown in Table 1–1.

Functioning as two-way communicators, nurses are able to maintain their roles as health providers while becoming therapeutic communicators—individuals who are able to find out what clients are hearing and understanding. These tasks require more time and effort, but they also can save needless suffering by both clients and nurses. Two-way communication is generally more effective than one-way communication, yet many nurses who understand this principle continue to perform many communication tasks as one-way communicators.

What follows is a list of reasons why nurses may use one-way communication though they believe in a two-way model.

- The communicator controls one-way communication.
- One-way communication can take place more easily while doing something else. Full attention to the recipient is not always necessary.
- Nurses feel under pressure to do a lot of tasks. Two-way communication may take away from other important aspects of client care.

Can you think of others?

EXERCISE IN ONE-WAY AND TWO-WAY COMMUNICATION

Pair up. One partner will be A, the other will be B.

1. Both A and B will (individually) think of two "nursing procedures" (or anything else) that have five steps.
2. Both A and B then write down their own procedures without showing them to each other.
3. A then reads the five steps in procedure one to B two times without any questions from B (one-way).
4. B then tells A what the steps are to the best of B's memory.
5. A then reads each step in procedure two to B and asks for questions or feedback after each step (two-way).
6. B then tells A the steps in procedure two to the best of B's memory.
7. Switch "roles" and re-do steps 3–6.
8. Discuss differences between the one-way and two-way communication sequences for both the "sender" and "receiver."
9. Discuss how you can improve client education through two-way communication.

Two-way communication is not always better than one-way communication. There are circumstances under which one-way communication is appropriate (like telling people the building is on fire). Furthermore, it may not, in certain circumstances, be possible to have immediate feedback and two-way

---

TABLE 1–1. COMPARISON OF ONE-WAY AND TWO-WAY COMMUNICATION

	One-Way	Two-Way
Ease	Easy	Difficult
Control	Sender	Sender and receiver
Feedback	None	Maximum
Flexibility	None required	Sender needs to be able to change according to receiver's feedback
Role of nurse	Teacher, evaluator	Therapeutic, corrective
Ways of determining understanding	Tests, long-term	Immediate

communication, as in the case of a comatose client. Another alternative which falls in between one-way and two-way communication is called "limited two-way communication" or "one-way communication with a feedback loop." In such a communication sequence there are specified limits or methods for feedback, such as question-and-answer periods. However, in many situations, the nurse can have a strong influence in facilitating two-way communication.

Context and the Interactive Nature of Communication

A component of the communication process that is not included in the model presented on page 6 is the setting or *context* in which the interaction occurs. Context is part of the title of this book and is a term which is used to mean the *total* situation or environment; in other words, context incorporates elements in the physical environment (e.g., noise or location), the psychological environment (e.g., feelings and attitudes), and the social environment, focusing on the relationship between the sender and the receiver. One cannot accurately interpret communication behavior without including these three aspects of the environmental context.

A key issue in all communication models is the linkage between the message and the receiver. In the case of a verbal message, all words have multiple meanings and all persons are unique. Therefore, a correct interpretation of the message is of prime importance. Problems arise when what persons *intend* in their communication differs from the actual outcome of that communication. The following incident serves as an example:

Mrs. Hart is scheduled to have an abdominal perineal resection and a colostomy. Her tests indicate cancer of the sigmoid colon. The oncology nurse (Miss Peck) has visited Mrs. Hart and explained exactly what is involved in the operation and what the colostomy will mean in terms of her life style postoperatively. On the evening before the operation, the nurse is expecting to give Mrs. Hart "saline enemas until clear." The dialogue that follows records the interaction that takes place (via the auditory channel) between Mrs. Hart and the nurse.

Miss Peck enters Mrs. Hart's room carrying treatment tray for saline enemas.

Mrs. Hart:	You're not giving that to me!
Miss Peck:	You are to receive saline enemas according to your orders.
Mrs. Hart:	Not me, you've made an error!
Miss Peck:	Mrs. Hart, you seem upset. It's not easy for you.
Mrs. Hart (distraught):	The other nurse told me I would have irrigations to regulate the colostomy *after* the operation, not before.
Miss Peck:	I think I understand where the confusion is—let me explain why the saline enemas were ordered.

In this situation, the nurse, Miss Peck, did not actually explain *what* was happening or *why* it was happening when she entered the room. The intended communication, which was nonverbal, was not interpreted correctly by the receiver, Mrs. Hart, who was to receive the saline enema. Miss Peck, however, was able to decode accurately the client's message and was able to clarify the purpose of the procedure.

In many situations, clients are reluctant to show their fear or concern with their illnesses, and choose to remain silent. In such cases, nurses really have three choices: to tell clients exactly what is going on, to say nothing, or to try to distract patients with reassuring clichés. Reassuring clichés create the highest level of stress: *it is better to say nothing* rather than give a false sense of reassurance. The healthiest approach, however, is created when the clients are given specific information in order to be prepared regarding their medical condition and progress (Roberts, 1986).

The interaction which occurred between the nurse and client regarding the saline enema procedure demonstrates a continuous, changing process or *interaction* in which the sending and receiving of messages occurs over a period of time. Each message affects the receiver. Both participants in the interaction continuously respond to each other, having been affected by the previous message sent.

COMMUNICATION THEORETICAL FRAMEWORK

Watzlawick, Beavin, and Jackson (1967) have provided the framework for communication theory in this book. Several basic axioms or principles of communication are presented in Chapter 2 of their book, *Pragmatics of Human Communication*. Each axiom examines communication as a range of behaviors rather than an isolated phenomenon. These axioms are briefly presented here and will be discussed more indepth in latter sections of this book.

1. *One cannot not communicate.* There is no such thing as noncommunication behavior; all behavior has message value. Activity, inactivity, and even silence can convey a message. Clients who do not respond verbally are conveying a message, and nurses can choose how to respond to the unresponsive client, including "not" responding or responding nonverbally (without words, using gestures, facial expressions, and so forth). Nurses cannot *not* respond. Finally, once the message has been sent, it is impossible to retract it. All communication is irreversible.
2. *Every communication has a content and relationship aspect such that the latter classifies the former and is therefore a metacommunication.* A communication sequence conveys a message, but at the same time implies a relationship structure between the two persons communicating. Watzlawick et al. refer to these two aspects as the "report" and "command" aspects respectively. The report aspect is the content of

the message; the command aspect refers to the way in which the message is received or the sender's view of his or her relationship with the receiver. How the communicators relate to each other is usually not on a conscious level; the relationship can be expressed verbally, nonverbally, or not at all. For example, in the case of Mrs. Hart:

Mrs. Hart: You're not giving that to me!
Miss Peck: You are to receive saline enemas. That's an order.

The last sentence, "That's an order," is a communication *about* the communication (also called a *metacomment*) and tells you something about the nature of the relationship between the sender and the receiver, namely, that Miss Peck felt she was in control of the contextual situation. In addition, the *way* in which the message was communicated (using nonverbal gestures or voice pitch) by Miss Peck to the client would influence the next response in this interaction. This relationship aspect is one feature of "communication about communication" and is called *metacommunication*.

3. *A series of communications can be viewed as an uninterrupted series of interchanges.* There is no discrete beginning or ending to a series of interchanges. In addition, one brings his or her totality of all past experiences to any communication interaction. Furthermore, the communication situation affects future communication as well.

   Watzlawick et al. note that there is an action-reaction chain of events in a communication series of interchanges. Consider the implications of a common reaction to clients who are chronic complainers (especially if there is a shortage of staff), that is, ignoring them. This in turn sets up a continuous cycle of events; clients complain, nurses ignore, clients respond by complaining further, and nurses react again by withdrawing from the situation. We have all had this experience at some point in our nursing careers. You may also think of situations in your own families or with friends in which you or others have unwittingly set up an unwanted "communication chain reaction."

4. *All communication relationships are either symmetrical or complementary, depending on whether they are based on equality or inequality.* Symmetrical relationships occur in interactions where the two partners in the dyad are considered as equals, such as two close friends. Complementary relationships, on the other hand, are those in which one partner in the dyad is "superior" to the other, such as parent-child or teacher-student relationships. It is obvious that communication is interpreted differently depending on the relationship the sender has with the receiver. There are a series of interesting questions and issues based on the relationships between senders and receivers, including nurse-nurse, nurse-client, and nurse-physician. The second section of this book deals with role relationships and will cover these areas in detail.

**EXERCISE IN COMMUNICATION
(WATZLAWICK'S PRINCIPLES)**

Break up into pairs and have a conversation about school, your families, or any other topic. After a few minutes, ask yourselves the following questions:

1. Can you accurately report what the other person has said? (content)
2. Are you aware of the relationship of what was said to the way it was said? (relationship)
3. Can you describe your partner's gestures, facial expressions, and posture? (relationship)
4. Did you encourage further communication from your partner? How? Did your partner encourage further communication from you?
5. Did you ask questions when you did not understand what the person was trying to communicate both in content and feeling?
6. Did you interrupt when your partner was talking? If you did, what led you to do so?
7. Did your talking together bring a positive feeling between you?

NURSING THEORETICAL BASE

Peplau (1952) was the first nursing theorist to present a theoretical nursing model based upon the interpersonal process. She defines nursing as a therapeutic interpersonal process consisting of actions that require participation between two or more individuals. Vital to this process is clear and supportive communication, which Peplau characterizes by *clarity* (when the meaning is understood and agreed upon by both sender and receiver) and by *continuity* (when the nurse picks up on threads of conversation that the client offers in the course of conversation). Both of these principles result in nurses' understanding clients' needs from the client's perspective. For example, Peplau believes that clients should participate in their own care and that the nurse-client communication process is basic to this participation. She encourages nurses to use nondirective techniques such as open-ended questions, clarification, and validation. (See Chapter 5 of this book for a discussion of related skills.) In addition, she believes that nonverbal behaviors are an integral part of communication. (See Chapter 4 for a discussion of nonverbal behavior.)

King (1981) supports and builds upon Peplau's framework. The theoretical concepts presented in her book, *A Theory for Nursing,* are also integrated into this book. An essential element of King's theory concerns the interactions that occur between the nurse and the client. An interaction, King postulates, is a process of perception between the person and environment (which in nursing is with nurses and other health professionals) represented by verbal and nonverbal behaviors that are goal directed (Parse, 1989). If goals are attained, effective nursing care will occur. King's theory is person-focused; persons are "open systems" interacting with the environment. She proposes three dynamic interacting systems, each of which is on a different level of abstraction—personal systems, interpersonal systems, and social systems. Selected concepts (see the following) are presented for each level and are covered in subsequent chapters of this book.

Personal systems (individuals)	Perception, self, body image, growth and development, time, space
Interpersonal systems (groups)	Role, interaction, communication, transaction, stress
Social systems (society)	Family systems, religious or belief systems, educational systems, work systems

Personal systems are individual; a nurse or a client as a person constitute a total system. *Intra*personal communication relates to this system level. Section I of this text focuses on the personal system.

Interpersonal systems consist of two or more individuals interacting with each other. Through perceptions of their environment and through verbal and nonverbal behavior, persons engage in interactions, some of which can lead to *transactions* that are purposeful interactions leading to goal attainment. *Inter*personal communication relates to this system level. Section II of this book focuses on interpersonal systems.

Social systems are composed of groups with special interests and needs who collectively can form an organization. For example, a hospital, a nursing group, or a family can constitute a social system. Sections III and IV of this book investigate communication behavior within a social system.

Definition of Nursing

Before proceeding further, it is necessary to define nursing. Consider the following definitions of nursing:

> Nursing is perceiving, thinking, relating, judging, and acting vis-à-vis the behavior of individuals who come to a nursing situation. A nursing situation is the environment in which the client and nurse interact for the purpose of setting mutual health related goals. (King, 1981, p. 2)

> Nursing is the diagnosis and treatment of human responses to actual or potential health problems. (ANA Statement, 1980)

Each of these generally accepted statements has two components, a concern with the medical or health-related condition *and* a concern with the client's reaction to the condition. Nursing is thus concerned with *reactions* of individuals and groups to actual or potential health problems, as well as the health problems themselves.

Nursing is also a process in which nursing actions are carried out in a series of steps called *the nursing process*. The basic idea of this systematic methodology, is essentially a modification of the problem-solving method.

THE NURSING PROCESS

The nursing process provides the foundation for nursing practice. It is a step-by-step method of selecting an action or actions to reach a desired goal. The major common thread throughout the nursing process is communication; it is the primary tool through which the nursing process is applied. The nursing process can be subdivided into four phases: assessment, plan, implementation, and evaluation.

Assessment
The purpose of the assessment phase of the nursing process is to identify human responses to actual or potential health problems. There are two components within this phase: data gathering and diagnosing. Data gathering includes collection of data through such means as observation, the health history, the interview, a physical examination, and record analysis such as the problem-oriented medical record. Communication skills necessary for this component of the nursing process are discussed in Chapter 5 of this text.

The second component within the assessment phase of the nursing process is the formulation of nursing diagnoses—the responses to actual or potential health problems that nurses are accountable to treat; the nursing diagnosis is the result of the nursing assessment. While skills in communicating with clients are essential in this phase of the nursing process, the nursing diagnosis concept provides the *single most powerful communication tool to unite the nursing profession.* The common language inherent in a nursing diagnosis is thought of as a universal language understood by all nurses. The nursing diagnosis, based on subjective and objective data, sets the stage for the remaining steps of the nursing process—planning, implementation, and evaluation of nursing care.

Plan
The second phase of the nursing process includes setting priorities and goals *for* and *with* the client. The global long-term goal of nursing is health. However, both long- and short-term goals set in this phase are specific and unique to each individual. This phase includes goal setting as well as identifying the means to achieve and evaluate these goals. The most effective means of communicating the plan of care to all involved health personnel and promoting

continuity of care is the written care plan. Carefully written documentation and care plans spare the client unnecessary repetition in giving information and promote coordinated care.

Implementation

Implementation is the action phase of the nursing process. This phase draws heavily on interpersonal and communication skills. Effective use of these skills enhances the success of the action. These communication skills may be utilized with the client, coworker, and other nurses. While the focus is action, this action may be intellectual and interpersonal as well as technical (Yura & Walsh, 1987).

Evaluation

The fourth phase of the nursing process is evaluation, in which the nurse considers how well the client responded to the planned action. Were the goals accomplished? If the client, for example, received a pain medication, is the pain alleviated? Nurse-client interaction is necessary for ongoing evaluation; however, observation of nonverbal behavior is important as well. In some settings, interacting with the client includes the client's family as well.

NURSING ACTIONS AND DEGREES OF VISIBILITY

In order to highlight the relationships of nurse-client interactions it is possible to group all nursing actions into three major clusters: physiological, psychological, and socioeconomic (Brown & Fowler, 1971). These clusters have considerable "overlap" in real life situations (Fig. 1–2) and represent the totality of nursing behaviors required to meet the needs of the client.

Physiological nursing actions include attending to the most obvious physical needs of the client. *Psychological nursing actions* include any and all activities

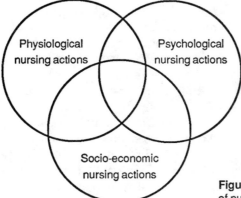

Figure 1–2. Representation of the three spheres of nursing action and how they overlap.

that affect (and aid) the emotional well-being of the client. *Socioeconomic nursing actions* relate to those nursing activities which address the client as a total person within the environment.

Of the three areas of nursing actions, psychological nursing actions are the most difficult to observe and measure. It is not easy to determine if what a nurse is saying has a therapeutic value for the client. For a moment, consider the case of Mary in the beginning of the chapter. How would you know from her reaction whether or not the nurse had *definitely* said the right thing?

One way of thinking about the three areas of nursing actions is to examine each in light of degree of visibility (Brown & Fowler, 1971), that is, what aspects of each area are most easily seen by others? As noted earlier, those actions related to the client's physiological needs are most easily defined as specific tasks and are most visible, while those related to psychological actions are the least visible. The latter are also most "person-oriented."

A nurse who is administering a tube feeding to a client is performing a nursing action related to a physiological need—maintenance of adequate nutritional status. This nursing action has a high degree of visibility. A nurse who is communicating with a client in a caring manner is performing a nursing action related to a psychological need. This nursing action has a low degree of visibility. That is, one cannot easily observe the outcome or the methods used to communicate in a caring manner. The assumption might be made by someone observing these nurses that the nurse administering a tube feeding is performing a nursing action to maintain the client's adequate nutritional status and that the nurse who is standing at the bedside talking to the client has finished with client care and wants to catch her or his breath before proceeding to the next client.

Table 1-2 summarizes the characteristics of high- and low-visibility actions (Brown & Fowler, 1971).

High-visibility tasks are easily seen by others, and are usually related to physiological functions. They can easily be broken down into steps, and require a high degree of psychomotor manual skill. At a less obvious level, they are easily routinized and are staff-centered. That is, high-visibility tasks focus on a nurse's activities and can therefore be controlled, monitored, and standardized. Similarly, the control and evaluation of these tasks is administered by power figures in the system, such as supervisors. Finally, high-visibility tasks have traditionally been the basis for reward (promotion, pay raises, and evaluation) in the hospital setting, which means that there has been a tendency to overvalue these tasks.

Alternately, low-visibility tasks are not easily seen by others, are usually related to psychological actions, require cognitive or affective skills as opposed to psychomotor skills, and cannot usually be broken down into identifiable steps. Because these tasks are highly interactive and dependent on immediate changes in the client, they cannot be routinized easily. They are also "client-oriented" for the same reason and are therefore less easily controlled by power figures, including supervisors.

TABLE 1–2. NURSING ACTIONS	
High-Visibility (Task-Oriented)	**Low-Visibility (Person-Oriented)**
Easily seen by others	Not easily seen by others
Require a high degree of psychomotor manual skill	Require high degree of cognitive/affective skill
Usually related to biological functions and processes of the individual	Usually related to psychological functions of the individual
Nonverbal	Verbal and nonverbal
Easily routinized—staff-centered	Not easily routinized—patient-centered
Can be easily broken down into steps— easy to teach	Cannot easily be broken down into steps that are identifiable and are difficult to teach
Controlled by power figures—nurse managers	Less easily controlled by high-status personnel
Traditionally highly rewarded in hospital settings	Traditionally not highly rewarded in hospital settings

A further point about low-visibility tasks is that their successful completion has not traditionally been rewarded or valued in the hospital setting. In part, the lack of reward follows from the difficulty of determining if a "good" job is, in fact, being done. At another level, the lack of reward is also due to the value judgment and philosophical orientation that stresses meeting the immediate physical needs of the client. Thus, areas such as counseling and health and family education are relatively recent arrivals in nursing curriculum. The growing evidence and research that points to the importance of less obvious activities (low-visibility tasks) in client care signal a change in nursing orientation that will strongly affect how nurses of the future function.

EXERCISE IN TASK VISIBILITY

Which of the following are high-visibility tasks? Which are low-visibility tasks? Which are both? Why?

1. Giving a bath
2. Counseling a client who is depressed
3. Showing a client how to administer insulin to himself
4. Talking to the client about her impending surgery
5. Taking a nursing history
6. Changing a dressing
7. Referring a "discharge patient" to the visiting nurse
8. Teaching a client crutch walking

Communication: High- and Low-Visibility Tasks

It is now obvious how communication relates to low-visibility and high-visibility tasks. Counseling, talking, and all such psychosocial activities require good communication, but what about fundamental nursing procedures? If you hold with the traditional value that high-visibility tasks are the only relevant ones for nursing, you might not find a use for this book. However, before closing the book forever, stop and think a minute. Put yourself in the client's place. Imagine yourself receiving care from a nurse. There are many ways in which the nurse communicates something to you. To put it another way, is it really possible for the nurse to *not* communicate?

Communication and High-Visibility Tasks. High-visibility tasks, as was discussed earlier, are marked by use of psychomotor skills, are usually related to physiological actions, and can be nonverbal. The communicative aspects of high-visibility tasks are not necessarily obvious but may have dramatic impact on the client, the nurse, and task completion *because* of their "hidden" or covert nature. Consider the following situation:

> A nurse was told to administer an intramuscular medication of vitamin K to a client. The medication was ordered to be given in the upper outer quadrant of the client's buttocks. The client, who had undergone surgery the week before, was uncertain what his status was. He thought the surgeons might want to operate on him again, but he wanted a second opinion before they "put him under." He remembered from the previous operation he had had a "preop" medication.
>
> The nurse came in and, thinking this was a simple physiological (high-visibility) task, started to turn the client over. The client saw the needle and physically resisted turning over. He also started to yell, "You're not going to give that to me!"

Clearly, a few words of explanation and reassurance (low-visibility tasks) would have made the procedure more acceptable to the client. Many nursing procedures for high-visibility tasks involve specific steps that include communication: namely telling what is going to happen and why. These steps are designed to prevent the problems the nurse encountered in the above example. How the message is delivered, and the client's physical, emotional, and verbal responses are important aspects of the communication process in high-visibility tasks.

There is also some communication in how the task itself is performed. For example, the nurse who is physically abrupt in turning a client over gives a very different message than one who is firm yet gentle. The response to the abrupt message will not always be obvious at that moment in time. You can be sure, however, that the client's attitude toward the abrupt nurse will be different from that toward the firm yet gentle nurse, with a variety of possible effects, including differences in compliance, demands, and personal anxiety.

Another area of high-visibility tasks that directly involves communication is history taking. Even though there may be a standard set of questions or data the nurse wishes to obtain, how the nurse asks the questions or communicates the questions will influence how much the client shares, how much concern is voiced, and even the client's mood. While history taking is primarily fact finding, communication and rapport building go on as well.

Communication and Low-Visibility Tasks. Low-visibility tasks generally focus on psychological functions. They are verbal and therefore have an "obvious" relationship to communication or how the message (information) is transmitted. At the same time, nurses, as well as other health professionals, often forget the impact even a small gesture, phrase, or motion can have on a client. The client is in a vulnerable, high-anxiety situation, either in a hospital, clinic, or at home, and will be affected strongly by almost everything the nurse says or does. This type of client interaction is described in more detail in Chapter 7.

Some authors go so far as to state that all psychological disturbances can be considered as problems in communication (Watzlawick et al., 1967). While this may or may not be true, the role of communication in both understanding and alleviating psychological distress is crucial. The term "therapeutic communication" is used to denote or point out communication sequences in which the purpose of the communication is to alleviate psychological distress. Ideally, the manner in which the communication is performed is caring, concerned, and empathic. While the specific knowledge needed to carry out therapeutic communication with severely disturbed clients is beyond the focus of this book, some of the skills covered in Chapter 4 will help in expressing care and concern for others more effectively.

A New Nursing Perspective and Communication. Today, nurses are shifting their emphasis from high-visibility tasks to an integrated approach that combines low-visibility skills with high-visibility skills. Qualified nurses do not perform a set of nursing tasks to the exclusion of the client's personal concerns. Nurses are finding out that often the best therapeutic communication can be carried out while they are performing high-visibility tasks.

One of the authors was recently talking to a neighborhood child, Michael, a 10-year-old. Michael had hurt his arm at school while playing football. He had an ace bandage put on his arm by the school nurse. The author, who was working on the book, asked Michael if he had any advice for nurses on how he likes to be treated. His first answer was "Be nice." When asked how the school nurse was nice to him, he replied, "She talked to me while she was putting on the medicine. She told me what would hurt and what she was going to do."

Although we were not at the "scene of the communication," we can speculate that the nurse used appropriate tones of voice, body gestures, and words to assure Michael that he would be all right. What the school nurse was in all likelihood doing was providing therapeutic communication (low-visibility, psychological action) *along with* administering first aid (high-visibility, physiological action) plus giving Michael health education information (low-visibility, socioeconomic and physiological action). The nurse, by combining high-visibility physiological tasks and low-visibility therapeutic communication did a good job with an upset 10-year-old. The ability to integrate the two areas is one we hope nursing students will develop in their nursing education and careers.

CONCLUSION

The purpose of this chapter has been to present a conceptual framework so that nurses can begin to integrate a basic knowledge of communication skills and the nursing process into their roles as health professionals. Communication models depicting the basic components of communication as well as how these components fit into the nursing process and nurse–client relationships are described. Nurses need to be aware of the content and relationship aspects of messages as well as the advantages of feedback to encourage two-way communication with others.

Nurse–client interactions do not occur in a vacuum; they occur in a health arena in which nurses are utilizing the nursing process to carry out their actions. These nursing actions can be contrasted in terms of visibility, with highly technical nursing actions at one end of the spectrum and communication interactions at the other end.

The unique role of the nurse is one that combines both high- and low-visibility actions; it is a role in which nurses minister to clients' physical and psychological needs. This is not an easy role, and much of the material presented in this text is designed to help students meet the challenge of assuming the demands of this professional role.

REFERENCES

American Nurses' Association. *Nursing: A social policy statement.* Kansas City, Mo.: American Nurses' Association, 1980.
Brown, M., & Fowler, G. R. *Psychodynamic nursing.* Philadelphia: Saunders, 1971.

King, I. *A theory for nursing.* New York: Wiley, 1981.

Laswell, H. *The structure and function of communication in society.* In L. Bryson (Ed.), *The communication of ideas.* New York: Harper & Row, 1948.

Parse, R. *Nursing science: Major paradigms, theories and critiques.* Philadelphia: Saunders, 1987.

Peplau, H. E. *Interpersonal relations in nursing.* New York: G. P. Putnam's Sons, 1952.

Roberts, S. L. *Behavioral concepts and the critically ill patient* (2nd ed.). Norwalk, Conn.: Appleton-Century-Crofts, 1986.

Watzlawick, P., Beavin, J., & Jackson, D. *Pragmatics of human communication.* New York: W. W. Norton, 1967.

Yura, H., & Walsh, M. *The nursing process* (5th ed.). Norwalk, Conn.: Appleton & Lange, 1987.

2 Communication Channels

By reading this chapter and participating in the exercises, students will be able to:

1. Categorize aspects of communication into visual, auditory, and kinesthetic components
2. Demonstrate an understanding of three levels of integration within each of three channels
3. Explain how thought relates to the major communication channels
4. Describe how language use relates symbolically to the major communication channels

Look at the following situation:

> A physician, nurse, and client were in the client's room: The physician was looking at the chart, the nurse was listening to the P.A. system, and the client was feeling some pain. The client moaned.
> "What did you say?" the nurse asked, turning to the client.
> "What seems to be the problem?" asked the physician.
> "I have pain!" stated the client, silently wondering why the physician and nurse were insensitive.

While the above incident is not dramatic, the communication between physician, nurse, and client was not very effective. Messages "sent" were not the ones received. One way of analyzing the miscommunication that took place in this example, and in communication in general, is to examine the channels that each person in the communication sequence used. Channels are the medium that "couple" or link the source of the message to the receiver. It is not always possible to isolate one channel from the others; however, effective use of and decoding of channel messages make for better communication. Nurses knowledgeable about channel use can detect systematic

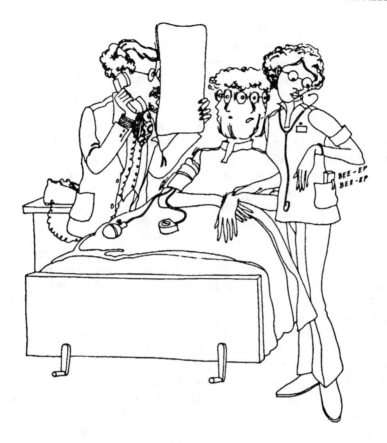

miscommunication and develop ways to improve communication with clients and coworkers.

COMMUNICATION IN THREE PRIMARY CHANNELS

One of the many interlocking components of the communication process is the channel or medium through which the message is conveyed. In communicating with a client, a nurse can notice the client's looks, clothes, manner of sitting, choice of words, tone of voice, voice volume, how he or she responds to the client, how it feels to touch the client, and even how the client smells. These are only a few of the possible things that could be experienced during a single communication!

One way of organizing all of this input is to categorize it into three general categories or channels: seeing (visual), hearing (auditory), and feeling (kinesthetic). These three represent major senses that all normal functioning human beings have to one degree or another. The content of a message may be important, irrelevant, immaterial, subliminal (i.e., the communicator is not aware of it), overlooked, or whatever, but in every nursing communication, there is visual, auditory, and kinesthetic input.

Within each channel, there are different levels of integration. That is, information that is seen, heard, or felt may be reported as it actually was seen, heard, or touched (Level I). The information may be reported in terms of observations, what the nurse got by really listening, or the nurse's feelings about a client (Level II). A third level integrates data from all three channels into the nurse's perceptions about the client (Level III). Level III builds on the information which was first sensed and was then integrated into one higher "full channel" level through the utilization of sensory input from all three lower channels (Levels I and II).

All experience begins with the taking in of information from the environment. Persons organize information through the use of their sensory systems and *perceive* the world around them. "Perception is a process of organizing, interpreting, and transforming information from sense data and memory" (King, 1981, p. 24). Perception is selective, based on past experiences and attending to what has been sensed (Level I), giving order and structure to the sensed data through one channel (Level II), and finally making associations from all three channels by interpretation of the data from Levels I and II. The three levels are presented in Figure 2–1.

The remainder of this chapter will focus on Levels I and II, since they are the most relevant to specific channel communication.

Many persons are unaware of the differences between levels of integration. Our past experience may have led us to state our observations, conclusions, or feelings, as if they were what we saw, heard, or felt. It is essential that nurses clearly separate these levels of integration so as to be able to assess the client's behavior, as well as to record findings accurately and to communicate effectively with clients. Imagine the following situation:

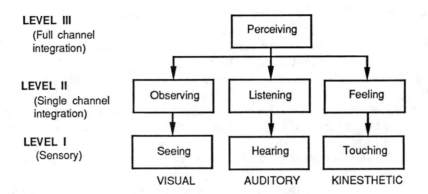

Figure 2–1. Communication levels.

A nursing student was asked by a nursing instructor to report on the condition of a client's wound:

"It's ghastly," the student said. "Also, it's oozing and the client is upset."

"How you feel is not relevant in this instance," replied the instructor. "Let's see if we can find out some information about the dimensions of the wound, the degree of infection, and the client's state of mind."

In this instance, the nursing student had to separate personal feelings from what was observed (Level II), as well as to categorize additional Level II data clearly; that is, the size of the wound and the degree of infection from how the client felt.

It takes practice to learn how to see and observe, to hear and listen, and to feel and react to clients or others in the environment. A good beginning is to master Level I, then move on to Levels II and III. An important point to emphasize is that functioning accurately at Level I (seeing, hearing, feeling) is as difficult as using Level II or III.

Although most persons selectively attend to a limited amount of information and have one channel they prefer to use, it is possible for the nurse to develop skill in all levels of integration in all communication channels.

The following sections examine the kinds of information to which nurses have access within each channel, as well as the ways they sense, perceive, and interpret this information.

The Visual Channel

In nursing communication, visual data can be interpreted rapidly to be given meaning. So, a shrug of the client's shoulders could mean "I don't know," a clenched fist may mean "I'm angry," and a man pacing back and forth in the waiting room of a surgical floor may mean "I'm anxious about the outcome of someone's surgery. One way of looking at visual information is to separate it into three levels: (1) what you *see*; (2) what you *observe*; and (3) what you *perceive*.

Seeing. Seeing is the least judgmental visual level. It is the closest nurses come to being a camera. Nurses are not, of course, merely cameras. They continuously interpret what they see without realizing it. For example, picture the room in which you ordinarily sleep. In one sense it is simply all of the hundreds of items that are found together (like a bed, blankets, floor, ceiling, light switch, dresser, etc.). Another way of seeing it is to view it as "my bedroom."

In communication, it is extremely important and difficult to be able to see things as they are. People are so prone to interpret visual information that a good deal of time is wasted being angry, upset, and so on over what is an "imagined" event.

One example of misinterpreting what is seen is given in the following story:

> While a nurse was changing a dressing on Mr. Kennedy's leg, she kept glancing at her watch. Mr. Kennedy was to go to the x-ray department in a half-hour and she did not want him to be late.
>
> "Why does she keep looking at her watch?" Mr. Kennedy asked himself. "She must be in a hurry to get the dressing changed so she can go have a coffee break with her friends."

Nurses sometimes find it difficult to report accurately what they have seen. The following exercise will help you begin to sharpen your "seeing powers."

EXERCISE IN SEEING

1. Pair up.
2. Sit across from your partner. Each of you will look carefully at your partner. Form a mental picture of your partner.
3. With your eyes closed, describe your partner's face, body, body position, and clothing.
4. Listen carefully as your partner tells you what you look like.
5. Describe how it felt to try carefully seeing another person, as well as to be carefully seen.
6. Discuss how your observations of clients are reflected in your clinical assessment.

Observing. The term "observing" implies that the nurse is operating at a higher conceptual level than just "seeing." The nurse is now making sophisticated interpretations about the client. Observation is hardly a new concept in nursing. Nightingale wrote in 1860:

> But if you cannot get the habit of observation one way or other you had better give up being a nurse, for it is not your calling, however kind and and anxious you may be. (Nightingale, 1969, p. 113)

Nurses primarily obtain information about clients in two ways: they *listen* to what clients tell them, and they *observe* the clients' objective signs and symptoms. Objective signs and symptoms are communicated primarily through nonverbal cues. Three objective signs in patients that are observed by experienced nurses without conscious thinking are skin color, breathing, and muscle tension. Skin color, the most obvious change, can vary from a flush to a cyanosis; breathing can vary with rate and rhythm; and muscle tension changes that are most noticeable around the eyes, the mouth, and the forehead between the eyes can be an indicator of relaxation or tension in the patient. In addition to these objective signs, most clients, especially if they are ill, tend to communicate feelings and attitudes *without* words.

Observing Body Language. In many instances, clients communicate their feelings to nurses through the use of body language. Understanding body language is to "see" how a person communicates through body actions. Nonverbal body language, also called kinesics, is socially learned in the same way one learns verbal communication. That is, people's body language differs due to unique family-rearing patterns or past experiences. Cultural variations in body language also exist. Just as a person has a unique way of talking, he or she has a unique pattern of kinesic behavior.

Body movement can be grouped under three types of activity: speech illustrators, symbolic gestures, and self-manipulative movements (Ekman & Friesen, 1984). *Illustrators* are nonverbal movements that accentuate or clarify verbal statements (Muldary, 1983). Touching one's body to indicate where the pain is and extending one's hands apart to show the length of a newborn are illustrators. The use and type of illustrators employed by persons usually indicates their ethnic background or culture. One commonly understood illustrator is the tendency by some cultural groups to "talk with their hands."

Symbolic actions are referred to as *emblems,* and have very specific verbal translations known to most members of a given culture. The most common examples of emblems are head nods meaning "yes" or "no" and shoulder shrugs meaning "I don't know." Although there are no universal emblems, certain emblems can unintentionally reveal some aspect of a message that a person is trying to conceal, such as the client who, when asked "How will you pay for your health care?," says nothing but shrugs her shoulders indicating she has no idea.

Self-manipulators, referred to as *adaptors,* are those movements in which one part of the body is doing something to another part. Examples of adaptors are rubbing one's nose, scratching one's head, or licking one's lips. Adaptors are the opposite of emblems; the person has little awareness of their presence. Many are thought to develop in childhood to satisfy needs such as nail biting (Blondis & Jackson, 1982). Adaptors are used by clients when the environment is hostile, tense, awkward, or stressful.

How do these nonverbal cues manifest themselves in nurse–client interactions so that the nurse can "see" the message? Three groupings of body language are often used in identifying nonverbal messages: facial expressions, eye contact, and posture.

Facial Expression. The most frequently used indicator of nonverbal body language is facial expression. Mehrabian (1981) contends that facial nonverbal cues make up over half of the total feeling message of a communication, feeling being either a specific feeling (e.g., joy, hurt) or more general (e.g., dislike or pleasure).

How, one may ask, is it possible that facial expressions that convey a message about how one feels make up over half of the total message? One reason is physical; the face is capable of many different movements because of its high degree of musculature, which permits sensitive changes in the forehead, eyebrows, eyelids, cheeks, nose, lips, and chin.

Much of the research on nonverbal behavior associated with facial cues has been conducted by Ekman and Friesen (1984). They found that there are facial "blueprints" for six of the major emotions: *surprise, fear, anger, disgust, sadness,* and *happiness* (Fig. 2–2). Each emotion can be further divided into a "family of expressions." For example, surprise has many variations: questioning, dumbfounded, dazed, slight, moderate, or supreme surprise.

It also seems that these six facial expressions can be accurately identified regardless of culture. Finally, it should be noted that facial expressions are brief in duration, varying from 1/5 to 1/8 of a second. It is easy to "see" why facial messages are frequently missed.

EXERCISE IN IDENTIFYING FACIAL EXPRESSIONS

Look at the six photos in Figure 2–2 and match one of the following six emotions with the appropriate photo: surprise, fear, anger, disgust, sadness, and happiness.

Answers to preceding exercises are:

1. Fear
2. Happiness
3. Sadness
4. Surprise
5. Anger
6. Disgust

Look at the first photo again. The emotion is that of a person experiencing fear. There is a distinctive appearance for fear—the *eyebrows* are raised and straightened, and drawn close together; the *eyes* are open and tense, the upper eyelids raised and lower eyelid tense; and the *mouth* is open but the lips are tense and may be drawn back tightly.

Fear is an emotion that nurses often see in clients who are ill. People who are sick fear harm will come to them, be it physical, psychological, or a combination of both. Physical harm may vary from something minor to actual life-endangering injuries. Psychological harm can also vary from minor insults or disappointments to extreme assaults on one's well-being (Ekman & Friesen, 1984).

Pain is another state frequently encountered by nurses. There is a distinct facial expression that accompanies pain. The facial expression of pain can be described as "brow lowering with skin drawn in tightly around closed eyes, accompanied by a horizontally stretched open mouth, sometimes with deepening of the nasolabial furrow" (LaReche & Dworkin, 1984, p. 1328). In addition, the facial expression of pain is fairly easily identifiable by health professionals when they are told to distinguish between it and other facial expressions in photographs (LaReche & Dworkin, 1984).

One of the difficulties in examining facial expressions of clients is that in many instances facial expressions represent a "blended" emotion. That is, two emotions (or even three) can occur simultaneously. For example, fear may occur with sadness, anger, disgust, or surprise.

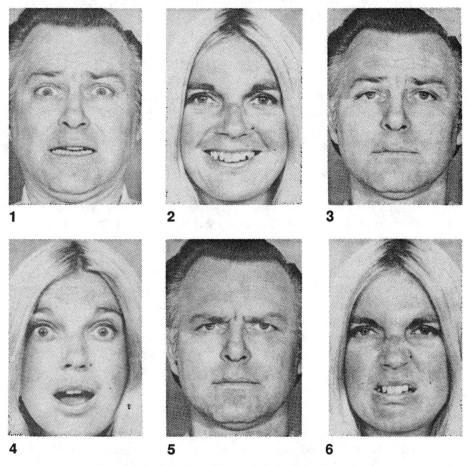

Figure 2–2. Ekman and Friesen's six universal emotions.

In addition, true feelings are often masked; persons learn to control and disguise their feelings so that what the nurse hears and sees is not always what the client feels. Facial expressions can give accurate cues as to the "real" client feeling.

Finally, a common difficulty faced by nurses is that they do not carefully attend to facial expressions, focusing solely on the content of the client's words. Consider the following situation:

Nurse:	How are you feeling today?
Client (facial expression is one of pain):	Fine.
Nurse (not noticing facial expression):	That's good.

In this interaction, the client responds to the nurse's inquiry by sending an incongruent message; in other words, his or her facial expression does not match the verbal message. However, the nurse, who is likely to be quite busy, may not be looking at the client when she is speaking and may miss the "obvious" inconsistency in the message. It turns out that people frequently do not watch each others' faces when talking but only look directly at each other as they finish speaking as a signal to the other that the communication has ended. Generally, facial expression is the most important indicator of feeling state. Another clue as to when the client is "hiding" feelings is a decrease in the number of illustrators, along with a related voice pitch level increase (Ekman & Friesen, 1984).

Research on facial expressions has implications for nursing. If nurses can understand facial "blueprints," they can correctly interpret the feelings of their clients and help them to cope with their response to illness. The first step for nurses, then, is to become aware of what clients' facial expressions are telling them by looking at their faces. A good place to start "looking" is with your family and friends.

Eye Contact. Of all the features of the human face, the eyes are the most important in transmitting messages and subtle nuances. Eye contact has been referenced in many different terms, such as "visual interaction," "eye signals," "gaze," and "mutual glance" (Exline & Fehr, 1982).

Almost any meaning can be conveyed from one person to another by such intricate movements as the length of glance, opening of eyelids, and squinting. Increased eye contact has been associated with an increase in positive feelings and attitudes indicating a greater liking between the sender and receiver (Mehrabian, 1981).

Clients can send many messages with their eyes. Often if they are stressed because of uncertainty relating to their health, they can totally avoid eye contact with nurses. Avoidance of eye contact can express other feelings as well—shame, fear, guilt, or low self-worth.

It is obvious that eye contact can be a highly sensitive form of communication. Consider the following example:

Mrs. Bigley, a new postoperative client, was to receive her first colostomy irrigation. As the nurse proceeded to explain the procedure, Mrs. Bigley was observed to avoid eye contact consistently. Because of her inability to establish eye contact, the teaching approach to Mrs. Bigley's colostomy care was not emphasized by the nurse, and the colostomy was irrigated without detailed explanation. The nurse's perception was that Mrs. Bigley was not yet ready to accept the teaching because of the psychological trauma of accepting the newly created defecatory exit. She waited until Mrs. Bigley seemed ready to accept instruction at a later time.

Mrs. Bigley avoided eye contact in this situation to maintain distance and prevent direct confrontation. The nurse concluded that avoidance of eye contact was the most valid indicator of the client's true feelings and changed the client care approach.

Nurses' use of eye contact deserves mention here as well. Persons in many Western cultures are taught not to stare at others; rather, eye contact interspersed with occasional averted gazes is more appropriate. Nurses, as well as other health professionals, are in a position to "put clients down" by staring at them without realizing they are doing so. One example of "staring" occurs in "medical rounds" in the hospital. Many clients find these rounds "dehumanizing," in part because the "team" of physicians, medical students, and/or nurses spend significant amounts of time staring at the client without communicating with him or her.

Posture. Posture is one area of client nonverbal behavior that is frequently overlooked by the nurse. For example, a client resting in bed can obscure his or her curled up, rigid and tense posture under the blankets.

Posture can give the nurse hints as to the client's emotional state. Is the client slouched over, or is he or she sitting rigidly or loosely? It is obvious that body behaviors such as posture can multiply meanings and communicate ambiguous messages; however, the body can be the key to understanding the real meaning of the message. When clients are attempting to deceive persons with whom they communicate, the body more than the face is a source of *leakage.* Leakage is a term used by Ekman (1983) to refer to a nonverbal act as revealing the true message that otherwise is being concealed.

Clients' posture can communicate an attitude toward the nurse. Posture can reflect a trusting and open attitude with arms at the side and a forward lean of the body, or a closed, defensive attitude with arms crossed or close to the body and the posture rigid and erect. Posture can also be a sign of how clients feel about themselves. Slumped shoulders and a bowed head are signs of depressed affect.

The posture of clients not only indicates their feelings of self-worth and how they feel about others, but how they feel physically. This is where nurses can be aware of the use of adaptors; for example, restless hand and foot movements, a wringing of hands, or picking at one's body. There is a high incidence of adaptors among clients who are anxious, nervous, ill and uncomfortable, and stressed, as in the case of hospitalized clients.

A client's general appearance can also give obvious clues as to how he or she feels. Men who are unshaven or women whose hair is uncombed may be communicating that they do not care or do not possess enough energy to care about their general appearance. Many clients lose interest in grooming self-manipulators. A sudden change in appearance is worth observing as a sign of health status change.

EXERCISE 1 IN OBSERVING BODY LANGUAGE

1. Pair up. Let one partner be *A*, the other *B*.
2. *A* picks one of the following emotions without telling *B* which one and expresses it by his or her facial expressions:

anger	joy
fear	boredom
surprise	impatience

3. *B* identifies the one *A* picked, and *A* then tells whether *B* is right or wrong. If wrong, tell the correct answer.
4. Repeat steps 2 and 3 three times.
5. Repeat the exercise but switch so *B* gets to express the emotion.
6. After the exercise is over, talk about it. Were there any expressions you could not "read" until you were told what they were? Did you notice any patterns in your partner's expressions of which he or she was not aware? You can also ask yourself, "What did I see that gave me the clue to observe that my partner was feeling anger, joy, or whatever?"
7. Discuss how client body language may lead you to conclude a client is suffering from pain, nervousness, or exhaustion.

The Auditory Mode

One way of thinking about all of the auditory aspects of communication is to imagine yourself sitting in a totally dark room talking to a person you cannot touch. Whatever goes on between the two of you will be completely auditory! Auditory aspects would include the words that are spoken as well as the volume, inflection, tone, pitch, rhythm, and speed of speech.

One way of organizing auditory input is to distinguish the content of words that are used (digital communication) from the tone, pitch, inflection, and speed of speech (analogical communication).

Nuances in auditory communication are often overlooked by nurses, as well as by others. The following exercise is designed to help you sharpen your awareness of how all of the analogical qualities of a message (tone, volume, pitch, rapidity of speech, etc.) can influence the impact of the message on the receiver.

EXERCISE IN AUDITORY AWARENESS

1. Pair up. One partner will be A, the other B.
2. A will say something that would normally be said to a client, such as, "How are you today?" B listens with eyes closed.
3. B then describes what A said in terms of the following:
   a. Speed of speech
   b. Volume (loudness)
   c. Pitch (how high, low the voice is)
   d. Inflection (how sing-song or "up and down" the words are)
   e. Rhythm of the words
4. Repeat steps 2 and 3 with roles reversed.
5. How do you feel when other people talk with an unusual cadence, pitch, or tone of voice?

Hearing. The same way that the first level of visual communication is seeing, the first level of auditory communication is *hearing.* Being able to identify accurately what you hear is a crucial step in nursing communication. It is also important to hear all aspects, not simply the words that are said.

EXERCISE 1 IN HEARING

1. Pair up. One partner will be A, the other B.
2. A says something A believes is true.
3. B mimics (tries to sound just like A did) the statement, reproducing A's speed of speech, inflection, pitch, volume, and rhythm.
4. Discuss how easy or difficult it is to mimic another.

EXERCISE 2 IN HEARING

1. Pair up. One partner will be A, the other B.
2. A says a simple statement.
3. B mimics A, but exaggerates *one* of the following:
   a. Speed of speech
   b. Volume
   c. Pitch
   d. Infection
   e. Rhythm
4. Repeat steps 2 and 3 with reversed roles.
5. Discuss how easy or difficult it was.

The above exercise is difficult and demonstrates that how the message is delivered has a tremendous impact on others. An awareness of one's own speech, as well as that of others, can be increased through practice in this exercise with a friend or with a tape recorder.

Listening. "To learn about a patient, one must talk little and listen a lot" (Brunner & Suddarth, 1980, p. 19). However, nurses, and persons in general, do not know how to listen.

Listening is often thought of as a passive or natural process, similar to hearing. Listening is actually an active, cognitive process. It is not easy to be an effective or "active" listener. The process of listening includes paying attention to both the verbal (spoken words) and the vocal (voice intonation, speed, pitch, and quality) aspects of the message. It requires sensitivity by the receiver to the message on a content as well as a feeling level.

One reason it is so difficult to listen may be the inability to concentrate; an effective listener may concentrate on the messages received for as long as 4 to 5 minutes before taking a mental break! During this brief "time out," the listener can rephrase the most pertinent points of the last few minutes. A sign of an effective leader in nursing (and other professions) is the ability to listen and then summarize what has been said.

Another reason for inability to be an active listener is the amount of interference or psychological noise that is present. Such distracting stimuli (noise, fatigue, boredom) are often present in health care settings, making it difficult for nurses to interact with clients.

There are many instances in which nurses communicate with clients by telephone, thereby rendering the visual channel ineffective. What happens if one is communicating with the client by means of the telephone and cannot see the client's nonverbal behavior? Two rules of thumb are: If what the client is saying is positive and the vocal expression negative, then the total message should be taken as a negative one; and, if the vocal expression is positive and the words are negative, the total message should be interpreted as a positive one. The next exercise will sharpen your listening awareness.

EXERCISE IN LISTENING

1. Record a conversation with a partner for 5 minutes using a tape recorder. The topic should be: "My own health habits."
2. Force yourself to listen to the *qualities* of the other's speech, that is, tone, speed, inflection, mannerisms, and so forth, as well as what is said.
3. Answer the following questions for yourself:
   a. When does the person's content (what he or she says) fit with how it is said? When does it not fit?

> **b.** What are the most striking aspect(s) of the other's speech? How does it (or the person) affect you? What assessment about the other would you make based on his or her speech?
>
> **c.** Can you figure out any *patterns* in the other's speech? (For example, is there a rhythmic sequence that indicates anxiety, a certain inflection to emphasize words?)

One of the mistakes often made in nursing communication is that meaning is assumed to be understood. That is, because two people are both nurses, they assume they know exactly what each other means by "care," "compliance," "following orders," or almost anything else. The following *true* story shows how a misinterpretation can occur in nursing communication.

Some beginning student nurses were working in a newborn unit. One of the infants had hydrocephalus, a condition in which the child's head is enlarged. The nurse in charge told the students, "Be sure to weigh and measure the head each day." To her surprise she returned to find the students trying to put the infant's head on a scale. What she had meant was "weigh *the baby* and measure the circumference of the head."

Rather than assume that all nurses should understand everything they hear, the effective nurse communicator has to work hard and listen carefully to "make meaning" or understand what others communicate.

EXERCISE IN MAKING MEANING

1. Pair up. One partner will be *A*, the other *B*.
2. *A* then makes a statement.
3. *B* then asks, "Do you mean. . .?" and finishes the question with *B*'s interpretation as to some of the underlying meanings behind *A*'s statement. For example, if *A* says, yawning, "I think it's late," *B* could ask, "Do you mean you're tired?"
4. *A* then replies, using only one of the following answers:
   Yes
   No
   Partially
   (*A* may be surprised by what *B* says in that it is a "yes" even though *A* was not aware of it in making the initial statement.)
5. *B* then asks, again, "Do you mean...?" until such time as one of the following happen:

> **a.** *B* gets a total of 3 "yes" answers or
> **b.** *B* gets so frustrated that she or he says to *A*, "What did you mean?" *A* then tells *B*.
> 6. Switch roles and repeat.
> 7. When the exercise is over, think or discuss how meaning can be misinterpreted and how there can be more meaning in what you say than you realize when you say it.

The Kinesthetic Modality

The third major modality or communication channel is the kinesthetic channel. The term "kinesthetic" refers to all aspects of communication relating to feelings. Touch and physiological responses to the environment are considered at the first level of integration (Level I). This level of touch is associated with nursing procedures and is primarily of a physical nature. It is referred to as "procedural touch." When physiological reactions are given a descriptive label or are called "feelings," they are at the second level of integration (Level II). This touch is primarily psychological in nature and is referred to as "caring touch." It is important to realize that what are commonly called "feelings" have a cognitive as well as an emotional component.

Touch. Physical touch is the most basic and primitive of all our senses. It is not only the most important (Montague, 1978), but the most personally experienced of all the sensations. Montague refers to the skin as "the oldest and most sensitive of our organs, our first medium of communication and our most efficient of protectors" (Montague, 1978, p. 1). The first exploration we have as human beings entering into the world is through the sense of touch; we are endowed with a sucking reflex at birth. Touch is the first sense to come into our conscious experience; we "feel" our way back into consciousness when coming out of anesthesia. Touch can function in a primitive fashion, such as an elderly person's foot shuffling to prolong the contact of the bottom of the feet with the walking surface in order to increase balance and coordination.

Our culturally learned rules about social touching need to be changed in the nursing role. Physical contact with clients is allowed and even required. While changing one's previously learned rules and guidelines about touching others is not easy, a touching gesture can carry a strong message of care and even help unlock a client's feelings. The following situation is a true story:

> Cathy, a beginning student nurse, was assigned to Mr. Moore, a 38-year-old male client with a diagnosis of severely advanced arteriosclerotic heart disease. Mr. Moore had a coronary bypass operation but was still immobilized and could not even sit in a chair without experiencing severe anginal pain. He was receiving pain medication p.r.n. While

Cathy was assisting Mr. Moore with his A.M. care, she felt a sense of frustration in not being able to communicate effectively with this man about his illness.

After Cathy finished with Mr. Moore's bath and was about to leave the room, she stood by the head of his bed for a few minutes and placed her hand on his shoulder. After a few moments of silence, Mr. Moore began to share his feelings about his family, his loss of his job, and his hospitalization. As Cathy stated later, the act of touching seemed to break down the last barrier to communication and close the distance between them.

An unplanned effective use of touch to which the client responded was utilized in the above situation. At the same time, a "touching" gesture may appear forward or misinterpreted by some clients. Others may like being touched and interpret it as caring on the part of the nurse. As in any form of communication, the nurse has to be sensitive to the client's responsiveness and reactions and be able to switch channels or otherwise adapt to the client's likes and dislikes.

Procedural Touch. Procedural touch is one of the most frequently used modes of communication within the health care system. Procedural touch is an essential aspect of nursing. It would be difficult to perform such nursing procedures as a bed bath or an injection without touching clients. Nursing procedures that involve touching the client invade the client's personal space, that is, the "bubble" that surrounds our bodies and defines the limits of space that are strictly "ours." One of the things that happens in the nurse–client relationship is that certain uses of procedural touch are expected and accepted within territorial limits of the client that might not be tolerated in other circumstances. The assumption of the client role allows for the invasion of his or her space by the nurse without question. All health professionals tend not to question the ill client's right to maintain his or her personal space when performing routine procedures (doctors probe and palpate, nurses lift arms and legs and rub backs).

Non-procedural touch, that is touch used to give emotional care and support, is more likely to elicit caring and empathic responses than procedural touch (Sweeney, 1982). Procedural touch used by nurses, however, can communicate caring as well.

Caring Touch. Caring touch integrates feeling with the act of physical touching and represents a higher level within the dimension of kinesthetic modality. In caring touch, the nurse conveys kinesthetic messages of concern and sympathy. A partial list of what is communicated through caring touch might include affection, emotional support, playfulness, and empathy. Some different types of touch gestures interpreted by both personnel and patients as "tender feelings" were hand touches, embraces, holding hands, arm in arm, and patient crying on nurse's shoulder (Farrah, 1979).

Caring touch can be more sensitive than procedural touch. A nurse who holds a client's hand or reassuringly pats the client's shoulder, communicates a message to the client. This message is basically one of caring and concern for the client, who usually responds in some manner, be it positive or negative, to the nurse's action. In caring touch, the nurse conveys kinesthetic messages of concern and empathy.

The use of "caring touch" by nurses involves a certain element of risk taking. It can be easily misconstrued by clients. Some nurses have difficulty using caring touch, especially those nurses who have not been accustomed to this sense of touch within their own families. The use of caring touch, however, is a skill that can be developed with experience. Nurses who work in extended-care facilities with elderly clients for long periods of time have ample opportunity to develop the use of "caring touch." This caring touch encourages a closeness, a sense of trust, and reassurance.

The therapeutic effectiveness of "caring touch" has been the subject of nursing research. There is ample evidence in the literature that the use of touch by nurses has a positive effect on patients. A basic tenet regarding the use of "caring touch" is that its effectiveness depends on the individual nurse's comfort in initiating the touch, as well as each client's comfort as the recipient of touch (Farrah, 1979).

The following exercise is designed to sensitize you to the ways nurses can communicate through touch.

EXERCISE IN TOUCH COMMUNICATION

1. Pair up. One partner will be *A*, the other *B*.
2. Sit so you can touch each other.
3. *A* then picks one of the following messages to communicate through touch (do not tell *B*):
   a. I'm angry with you.
   b. I'm anxious about touching you.
   c. I care (have empathy) for you.
4. *A* then touches *B* on the hand, arm, shoulder, or some other part of the body, and
   a. communicates the "touch message" *A* has picked *while*
   b. *A* says, "Hello _____, how are you today?"
5. *B* determines what *A* was communicating through the touch (*A* tells *B* what the answer was).
6. *A* tries two more touches with the same verbal message: "How are you today?"
7. Switch so *B* can try some touch messages.
8. What have you learned about touch? Discuss how you can convey caring messages to patients by touch?

Some of you will find this exercise easier to do with your eyes closed. When you talk about the exercise, answer the following questions:

- How much did you think about your touch messages?
- How aware are you of your own or other people's touch messages?
- How do you and others respond when two different messages are given verbally and by touch?

When you think about it, there are not many different "feelings." There are, however, an infinite amount of *kinds* of one feeling, such as love. A fairly complete list of feelings includes:

loneliness	sadness
hurt	disappointment
love	frustration
sexiness	fear
happiness	anxiety

While feelings are experienced by the individual, often the nurse responds to the client's feelings by having similar reactions. This sense of being in the "other's shoes" is called empathy and is an important tool in therapeutic communication, which is discussed further in Chapter 4.

Much of the material relating to sensory modalities is relatively new to nursing. The whole concept of communication channels and the system of psychotherapy based on it, neurolinguistic programming, provides nurses with a new set of communication skills the results of which can mean increased choices and flexibility for both the nurse and the client. As a result, nurses will begin to see, hear, and feel differently (Knowles, 1983).

Nursing research in this area is in the early stages. An increased knowledge regarding clients' use of preferred sensory systems could result in nurses' use of different therapeutic communication approaches. One study, for example, explored and documented preferred sensory systems used by clients under postsurgical stress. Preliminary findings showed that there was a higher use of kinesthetic motor (movement) and auditory channels, as well as the olfactory and gustatory channels; there was less use of the visual internal channel (mental images of one's self as opposed to the external visual channel, for example television). However, there seems to be no primary sensory system upon which people rely in order to cope with stress (Loomis, 1983).

THE USE OF LANGUAGE, CHANNELS, AND COMMUNICATION

The concept of communication channels has a wide range of applications. (See Bandler & Grinder, 1975, and Grinder & Bandler, 1976 for a therapeutic system based on principles of channel use; the following discussion is in part based on their system). Almost all communication can be analyzed by the three major channels. We can even break down how we think, how we feel, what we say, and the kinds of activities we like to do into visual, auditory, and kinesthetic components. For example, listening to the radio is obviously an auditory activity, although we may visualize images based on what we hear. Playing tennis or many other sports is a combination of visual and kinesthetic activities (if we have ever played doubles and our partner got angry with us for a mistake, we may have also found an auditory component as well).

Nursing communication is similar to all other communication in that all nursing communication can be broken down and analyzed by auditory, visual, and kinesthetic components. Imagine the following case:

You are given an assignment by your head nurse. Your instructions are to help pass out meals. The meals arrive, you read the names on the plates, and give the trays to the appropriate clients. Feeling you have done this quite well, you wait until all are finished, then quickly collect and stack up the trays. As you are stacking them up, something drops out onto the floor. You look at a set of dentures and go immediately to the head nurse, dentures in hand. "Don't worry," she tells you, "you see we know this happens. If you look inside the dentures you will find the client's name on them. Many older people don't eat with their dentures in. They place them on the tray. We have to be careful to watch after the client has finished, as well as before, to make sure they don't lose their dentures."

There are many ways to examine what happened in this imaginary series of communications and activities. From the communication channel view, a partial breakdown would be as follows:

- Auditory—you were *told* directions
- Visual—you successfully *saw* the names of the trays and matched them to the clients
- Kinesthetic—you *gave* the meals to the clients
- Kinesthetic—you *felt good* about doing the job, which may have lowered your level of watchfulness after the meals were passed out
- Visual—you *saw* the dentures fall out but did not *see* the name in the dentures
- Auditory—you *spoke* to the head nurse
- Auditory—the head nurse *told* you information and a visual strategy to watch carefully *after* the meal for future use
- Kinesthetic—you *gave* the dentures to the client

It should be stressed that this analysis is extremely basic. One could go even deeper and examine how you interpreted the instructions (did you repeat them to yourself or make a picture?), how you went about matching the trays to the clients, how you used the "feeling good" to relax your watchfulness after the meal, and how you processed the final information from the head nurse. All of this could have been done through the channels concept. It is thus possible to examine thinking, use of language, and many aspects of nursing process and communication through the concept of channels.

Thinking in the Three Major Channels

People rarely pay attention to how they think. They can usually tell you what is on their mind, what their secret hopes are, or what they want for Christmas, but most of them are not aware of *how* they think. By "how," we are talking about visual, auditory, and kinesthetic thinking, as well as the steps people go through to decide what they want for Christmas, what is on their mind, or, in the case of client–nurse communication, what the presenting complaint is. It can be quite important to understand how (not what) a client thinks, because the *process* of thinking and speaking may overlook important information that is essential to the client's care. An example will help clarify the last statement.

Suppose you are the nurse for a postoperative client. You come by and ask him, "How do you feel?" He thinks for a second and says, "Lousy." You pursue the point and discover that the client, when asked "How do you feel?" uses visual thoughts (he pictures himself) to decide how he feels. Furthermore, because it is difficult to "picture how you feel," he quickly (without being aware of it) pictures himself in bed, groggy eyed, in a hospital, and then compares this picture to one of himself playing golf and says, "Lousy."

Visual Thinking. When we think visually, we create pictures. If we imagine for a moment what our house or apartment looks like, we begin to get some sort of a picture of a building or rooms in our mind's eye. People who are very good visual thinkers can make mental lists of tasks to do, can picture each step in a nursing procedure, or can imagine how a certain size client will fit a certain size wheelchair.

These last examples show us some of the advantages of visual thinking (picturing). Visual imaging can also be useful in interpreting what a client or staff member is saying. In the case of the falling dentures, we could make a picture of ourselves looking at the trays after the meal and use that picture to remind ourselves to do it.

Information from hearing or feeling channels can also be visualized. If we have trouble listening or being responsive to feelings at a moment in time, this can help our understanding and communication. One way to visualize what a client is saying is literally to make the words go across our mind's eye like a typewriter. That way, we can "see" what is being said. If there are many "feelings" coming out, we can make pictures in our mind's eye of someone feeling those feelings. That way, we can "see what they mean."

Ideally, all nurses develop abilities to communicate and think in all channels. The following exercise is a simple way of sharpening your visual thinking processes.

EXERCISE IN VISUAL THINKING

1. Pair up. One partner will be *A*, the other *B*.
2. *A* then slowly describes a nursing procedure to *B*. The procedure should have between three and five steps. (Procedures like how to take a temperature, ambulate a client, or give a bed bath are fine.)
3. As each step is described, *B* pictures performing the procedure.
4. At the end of the description, *B* tells *A* how to do the procedure by thinking of each picture and describing what is there.
5. Repeat steps 2–4 with roles reversed.
6. Optional: Repeat steps 2–5 with a nine-step procedure.
7. Discuss how picturing may help you both prepare to perform a procedure, and as a review, what you have accomplished with a client.

Thinking in the Auditory Channel. In the same way that some people picture their thoughts, others think in auditory mode, primarily by subliminally talking to themselves.

Visual and kinesthetic information can be thought about in an auditory way simply by using words to describe the information. For example, when a nurse writes "patient slept well" on a chart, these nursing notes represent auditory thinking about what was observed. The nurse received the information through the visual channel and thought of appropriate words to use.

As nurses, we are aware of the extreme importance of being able to describe accurately or to find the right words for behavior and symptoms. Mistakes in auditory thinking can lead to confusion for both the client and the nurse. For example, a common nursing procedure is to obtain a "clean catch" urine specimen. Because of the nature of this specimen collection, the procedure must be explained (auditory channel) to the client and the client must "collect" the specimen. The client is instructed to wash thoroughly before voiding and then, while emptying the bladder, to "catch" the midstream portion of the voiding in a sterile container. This is sent to the laboratory for examination of microorganisms present in the urine. In order for the client not to contaminate the specimen, instructions are given to void the first and last parts of the urinary stream into the urinal or bedpan. As is obvious even in the explanation here, this is not an easy procedure to explain. Clients will often void the entire specimen into the bedpan because they did not "hear" the nurse, and the procedure must be re-explained and performed again. It might be far easier in this instance to demonstrate by a chart (visual channel), but many hospital procedures do not lend themselves to visual demonstrations.

EXERCISE IN AUDITORY THINKING (SELF-TALK)

1. Pair up. One partner will be *A*, the other *B*.
2. *A* then slowly describes a nursing procedure to *B*. The procedure should have between three and five steps.
3. As each step is described, *B* tells him or herself the step.
4. At the end of the description, *B* tells *A* how to do the procedure by first saying the steps over to him- or herself and then telling *A*.
5. Repeat steps 2 through 4 with roles reversed.
6. Discuss how self-talk can help you prepare to perform a procedure or evaluate what you accomplished with a client.

Thinking Kinesthetically. Although most people tend to use visual or auditory channels, some do think kinesthetically. Usually "feeling" thoughts are triggered by "feeling" words. If we began to think about the last time we felt really sad about something, we might find ourselves feeling sad: our breathing might change and our stomach might "feel a little sad." We could also be seeing the scene and hearing the words that were said, but because we are assessing kinesthetically, we will be feeling "feelings" or body responses.

EXERCISE IN KINESTHETIC THINKING

1. Say each of the following emotion words to yourself or out loud with "feeling":

angry	joyous
silly	rude
crazy	sentimental
sad	happy
sexy	

2. Think about how each "feels."
3. Discuss how your feelings on a given day may affect your assessment of a client.

It is also possible to think through the sense of smell. While we do not usually think in this mode, odors are often related to strong emotional experiences in the past.

Speaking in the Channels

Along with thinking in the modes, people's use of language can be related to channels. According to Bandler and Grinder (1975), who have developed a system of psychotherapy and have stated the use of modalities in communication most eloquently, the majority of people have a predominant mode; that is, they are primarily visual, auditory, kinesthetic, and occasionally olfactory in their use of language. For example, some people use a lot of phrases like "I see what you mean," "I need a clear picture," or "My view is." The key words here are *see, picture,* and *view.* They are all visual terms. The person using them can be considered a visual person.

Another person may habitually use phrases like "I hear you, Let's talk about," and "Listen to what I have to say." The key words for this person's major channel are *hear, talk, listen,* and *say.* These words are all auditory, that is, they relate to hearing. A person using predominantly phrases like these is likely to be an "auditory" person.

A third possibility is the person who uses phrases like "My feeling is, I'm in touch with," or "I can't grasp his meaning." The key words in this instance are *feeling, touch,* and *grasp.* All of these words are kinesthetic. They all relate to "feeling." A person who uses phrases like these will be referred to as a "kinesthetic" person.

According to Grinder and Bandler (1976), many people primarily use one channel for communication. That is, they use either visual, auditory, or kinesthetic terms to express themselves. In addition, they are likely to appreciate communication from others in their own channel. What this suggests is that the effective nurse communicator needs to be "fluent" in all channels and capable of switching to the client or other health professional's channel to be understood, as well as to create empathy and rapport. The following section is designed to facilitate the development of channel-specific language.

Visual Language. Several "visual" terms have been given above. A good list of visual terms includes:

television	perspective	map
see	demonstrate	graph
clear	show	viewer
picture	design	read
view	chart	review
appear	watch	preview
look	reflect	seem
seemingly	visionary	appearance
clearly	overview	vision
focus	clairvoyant	

Many people have some familiarity with these words. Often, these words appear in phrases like "I read your mind," "look out," "I see where you're at," and "show off." They can all be used to convey or make meaning. Some people (low-visualizers) rarely use them to describe their experiences. Others (high-visualizers) may use them exclusively. The following exercise is designed to help develop and recognize the abilities we have as a speaker of visual images. "See" how you do.

EXERCISE IN MAKING VISUAL MEANING

1. Read the first nursing-related statement in list 1 below.

List 1	List 2
a. I need to know more about your health history.	a. Let's *focus* a bit more on your health history.
b. Where is the pain?	b. *Show* me where the pain is.
c. I understand you.	c. I *see* what you're saying.
d. I do not understand you.	d. I don't *see* what you mean.
e. I hope you are comfortable here.	e. I hope everything *seems* well.
f. What is your problem?	f. What *seems* to be the problem?
g. Did the doctor communicate what is wrong?	g. Did the doctor *review* your diagnosis?
h. How are you feeling today?	h. How does everything *seem* today?
i. I need some information about your family?	i. Give me a *picture* of what your family is like.

2. Then, say the *same* thing, only use a *visual* image to convey your meaning.
3. Compare your answer to the statement in list 2 to see if you matched or were close to the one we give. (There are more options than the ones in list 2. The ones we give are simply to help you if you cannot come up with one of your own.)
4. Continue down the rest of the list, comparing your answers with ours.

The more we practice statements such as those listed above, the more likely we are to communicate clearly with a visualizer. In a very important way, being able to speak in the other person's channels is like talking in Spanish to a resident of Mexico. We stand the best chances of being understood when we speak the client's language. If we *see* the meaning and will *review* this point several times, we will be more effective visual communicators.

Auditory Language. All auditory language relates to hearing. A good list of auditory terms is:

auditory	resound	thunder
hearing	speaker	melody
hear	singing	spoken
read	loud	roar
speak	say	whistle
music	tell	sound
perform	ear	soft
radio	aural	sing
words	record	noise
blast	concert	

Many of these words are part of phrases or slang that are commonly used in American culture. "I hear you," "sounding board," "tell him off," and "speak your mind" are only a few. As was the case for visual expressions, each conveys its own special meaning. They will be particularly useful if the person with whom we are speaking is a "high-auditory" that is, the person uses a lot of auditory words and is sensitive to the nuances of auditory communication.

As was the case for visual language, auditory language can be used to make meaning out of language in other channels (sentences using seeing or feeling words), as well as language without a specified channel. One example from common nursing communication is as follows. Suppose you went to a client's bedside and wanted to ask about the operation. In a visual channel you might say. "What was your *view* of the operation?" An auditory translation would be "*tell* me how the operation went." It is surprising how some clients will respond to one of these more easily than the other. (Some clients will respond best to a "kinesthetically phrased" question—see below.)

The following nursing-related statements are similar to those translated into visual language earlier. This time, translate them into auditory language that gives the same meaning as the original statement. After you have made your translation, compare your answer to the ones on the right side of the page.

List 1	**List 2**
I need to know more about your health history.	*Tell* me more about your health history.
Show me where the pain is.	*Tell* me where the pain is.
I understand you.	I *hear* what you are saying.
I do not see what you mean.	I can't *tell* what you mean.
Are you comfortable?	How would you *say* you feel?
What seems to be the problem?	*Tell* me what the problem is.
Did the doctor communicate what is wrong?	Did the doctor *say* what the problem is?
How are you feeling today?	*Say,* how are things here today?
Give me a picture of what your family life is like.	I'd like to *speak* to you about your family. How does that *sound*?

Kinesthetic Language. Kinesthetic words and phrases refer to feeling, touch, and other aspects of kinesthetic senses. They are often combined with visual or auditory connotations. A list of kinesthetic terms would include the following:

sadness	itch	felt
touch	pain	fear
feel	anger	smooth
hostility	joy	soft (also auditory)
grasp	glad	scratch
handle	move (also visual)	painful
rough	blast (also visual or auditory)	hurt
hard	touchy	love

Many slang expressions use feeling words. Some familiar ones include "go with the *feelings*," "it's *hard* to tell," "caught between a rock and a *hard* place," and "on the *run*." Several of these are combined with terms from other modalities.

Along with high-visualizers and people who are primarily auditory in language use, some people have a great deal of skill in using kinesthetic language. While one may hesitate to call them the "feelers" because of how that can be misinterpreted, they can be considered as high-kinesthetics.

The following exercise is similar to the previous translation exercises. Translate the nursing communication in list 1 on the left of the page into kinesthetic sentences. Compare your answers to those in list 2 on the right side. Remember, there is more than one way to say something in a "feeling manner."

List 1	**List 2**
I need to know more about your health history.	I need to get a *feel* for your health history.
Show me where you think the pain is.	Where do you *feel* the *pain* is?
I hear what you are saying.	I *feel* I *grasp* your meaning.
I do not understand you.	I am not in *touch* with your meaning.
I hope that everything seems right.	I hope you *feel comfortable.*
What is the problem?	What do you *feel* is wrong?
Did the doctor tell you the diagnosis?	Did the doctor tell you what he *felt* was wrong?
How does everything seem today?	How are you *feeling?*
I need some information about your family history.	I need some *hard* facts about your family.

Some of these statements might be *hard* to say. You are encouraged to practice them as a challenge.

Olfactory Language. Few if any of the readers of this book will use olfactory words as their major channel of communication. Words that suggest smell or taste (the two are closely related), however, can quickly remind us of emotions. The following is a list of olfactory and taste-related words:

smell	mildew	sugary
scent	baking	aroma
taste	fumigate	smelling
spit	tasteless	moldy
sweet	odor	acidic
pungent	tangy	perfumed
aromatic	bitter	odorless
stuffy	salty	sniff

Olfactory terms are also commonly used in the following expressions. As an exercise, translate each into the channel noted at the end of each statement. Compare your answers to those we have supplied in list 2.

List 1	List 2
Something smells fishy. (make it visual)	Things do not *look* right. (visual)
The food is bland. (make it auditory)	I *hear* the food stinks. (auditory)
She sure is saccharine sweet. (make it feeling)	It is *hard* to believe that she's that nice. (kinesthetic)
This is bitter medicine to swallow. (make it visual)	This *seems* awful to accept. (visual)
What's cooking? (make it auditory)	What's the good *word*? (auditory)
That joke is so old it's moldy. (make it feeling)	That joke is so old it *feels* corny. (kinesthetic)
That was a tasteless comment. (make it visual)	In my *view*, that comment was inappropriate. (visual)
I'm just sniffing around. (make it auditory)	I'm just *listening* to what everyone is saying. (auditory)
Spit it out! (make it feeling)	Say what you *feel* about the matter. (kinesthetic)

Channel-Specific and Channel-Nonspecific Language
So far, much of the discussion has focused on language that suggests a channel. For example, "see" suggests the visual channel, "hear" the auditory channel, and "feel" the kinesthetic channel. However, not all words suggest a channel. That is, there are many words that are not specific to any channel. They are good to use when one is not sure "what channel" the other person is on. A partial list of verbs or action words *without* a specified or implied channel is as follows:

think	distinguish
decide	wonder
sense	like
conclude	understand

As you think about it, you can *think, decide, wonder,* or do any of the above terms in *any* of the channels if you put your mind to it. The important distinction here is to separate words that imply one channel from words that do not directly indicate any particular channel.

CONCLUSION

The purpose of this chapter has been to highlight the differences inherent in the three major communication channels. The relationship among the channels of communication when we think, speak, and feel has been presented. Channel preferences and the utilization of one major, predominant channel have been emphasized throughout.

What should have become apparent to you in reading this chapter is that emotions or the way one feels are powerful forces in the communication process. One's feelings will be expressed one way or another. If emotions are denied an outlet through one means, for example verbal expression, they will find another outlet such as body language. Keen, accurate, precise observational skills are vital for a minimal competence level in professional nursing. Finally, when sending a message, tune into the client's primary channel. This might require attending to a channel you do not normally use.

REFERENCES

Bandler, R., & Grinder, J. *The structure of magic. I.* Palo Alto, Calif.: Science and Behavior Books, 1975.

Bandler, R., Grinder, J., & Satir, V. *Changing with families.* Palo Alto, Calif.: Science and Behavior Books, 1976.

Blondis, M. N., & Jackson, B. E. *Non-verbal communication—Back to the human touch* (2nd ed.). New York: Wiley, 1982.

Brunner, L. S., & Suddarth, D. S. *Textbook of medical-surgical nursing.* Philadelphia: Lippincott, 1980.

Ekman, P. (ed.). *Emotion in the human face* (2nd ed.). New York: Cambridge University Press, 1983.

Ekman, P., & Friesen, W. V. *Unmasking the face* (2nd ed.). Englewood Cliffs, N.J.: Prentice-Hall, 1984.

Exline, R. V. & Fehr, B. J. The assessment of gaze and mutual gaze. In K. R. Scherer, & Ekman P. (Eds.), *Handbook of methods in nonverbal behavior research.* Cambridge: Cambridge University Press, 1982.

Farrah, S. *The nurses' reported use of touch.* Master's Thesis (unpublished), University of Illinois, 1979.

Grinder, J., & Bandler, R. *The structure of magic II.* Palo Alto, Calif.: Science and Behavior Books, 1976.

King, I. *A theory for nursing.* New York: Wiley, 1981.

Knowles, R. D. Through neurolinguistic programming. *American Journal of Nursing,* 1983, 83(6), 1011–1012.

LeReche, L., & Dworkin, S. F. Facial expression accompanying pain. *Social Science in Medicine,* 1984, 19(12), 1325–1330.

Loomis, M. *Linguistic analysis of verbal communication.* Paper presented to the Midwest Nurses Research Society. Iowa City, April 11, 1983.

Mehrabian, A. *Silent messages* (2nd ed.). Belmont, Calif.: Wadsworth, 1981.

Montague, A. *Touching* (2nd ed.). New York: Harper & Row, 1978.

Muldary, T.W. *Interpersonal relations for health professionals: A social skills approach.* New York: MacMillan Publishing Co., 1983.

Nightingale, F. *Notes on nursing.* London: Dover Publications, 1969.

Sweeney, S. H. *Student nurses' empathic touch and emotive perception.* Master's Thesis (unpublished), University of Illinois, 1982.

3 Communication Styles

By reading this chapter and participating in the exercises, students will be able to:

1. Identify the following aspects of communication styles: openness, person-task orientation, self-disclosure, acceptance, defensiveness, and congruence
2. Understand the concepts of self-worth and stress
3. Contrast the communication styles of blaming, placating, superreasonableness, irrelevance, and congruence
4. Translate incongruent communication into congruent responses

All human interactions include some form of communication. In addition, these interactions are characterized by unique communication styles utilized by individuals in the process of sending and receiving messages. What exactly is a communication style? In one sense we all have our own style of communicating; each of us is unique, with different ways of communicating and interpreting the same message. If we stop to think about it, we could no doubt describe the way we communicate in so many words or phrases. The following words or phrases have been used to describe the communication styles of different people at various moments in time:

talks too fast	talks slowly
gestures a lot	undemonstrative
dominates discussion	submissive
kids around	serious
passive	aggressive
scattered	straightforward
open	closed
listens	does not listen

One's communication style can vary according to the situation. For example, some nurses may be submissive with a physician and then turn around and be dominant with a client. Clearly, style is a function of abilities and strategies, as well as the context in which the communication takes place.

One way to think about our communication style is to examine it in light of several concepts or dimensions. The following six dimensions are commonly used to analyze communication styles: openness, person-task orientation, self-disclosure, acceptance, defensiveness, and congruence. Each dimension can be conceptualized as a continuum, with various degrees or points along which we may place ourselves. Although there are several dimensions that have a clear "healthy" position (such as being open, accepting, and nondefensive), there is still no single "magic formula" for an effective communication style in all of these. As you read the following discussion about these six dimensions, think about circumstances under which you would want to exhibit varying degrees of each dimension.

Openness

The concept of openness is commonly used to describe communication styles. We often hear another person described as "really open." Similarly, the other end of the openness dimension is characterized by the statement, "He's pretty closed to praise or criticism." Openness is related to the ability to listen, understand, and accept differences and criticism.

Openness on the part of the nurse encourages the client to take initiative and think through problems (Murray & Zentner, 1989). Whether or not new information can be added to an existing communication system will determine its openness.

At a practical level, the idea of openness is not clear. In order to adequately understand another's openness, it is necessary to ask the following questions: "Open to what?" and "Open to whom?"

"Open to what?" refers to kinds of messages you, as a nurse, are open to receive. A short list of types of messages includes:

- Information (e g., how to perform a procedure)
- Praise (e.g., a compliment)
- Criticism (e.g., a complaint)
- Inquiry (questions)
- Corrective feedback (criticism and suggestion)

To which of these are you most open? That is, which are easiest for you to listen to and accurately understand about yourself? Which are the most difficult for you?

"Open to whom?" refers to the role relationship in which nurses and the other person exist. Some examples include: physician–nurse, nurse–nurse, nurse–aide, nurse–client, and nurse–family member. (See Section II for a much more extensive explanation of roles and nursing communication.) Although individuals differ, people in general respond differently in terms of openness to communication from superiors, peers, or subordinates. For example, students react differently to criticism from a teacher (superior), a classmate (peer), or someone in the class behind them (subordinate). In thinking about how open we are to various kinds of messages, we can examine our reaction to the source (superior, peer, or subordinate).

Person–Task Orientation

Another way of describing a person's communication style is person–task orientation (Blake et al., 1981). The idea behind this dimension is that people vary in their focus on the person and the task. A common description for some people is "totally task-oriented." Others may be highly person-oriented. People can be high on both, low on both, or high on one and low on the other. The person–task orientation can also change depending on the situation. Although not technically a style, your person and task orientation will affect how you communicate and what information you attend to in communicating with others.

EXERCISE IN RATING YOUR PERSON–TASK ORIENTATION

1. Pair up with a partner.
2. First rate yourself in general as low, medium, or high on the following two dimensions:

Person	Task
Low: Little or no attention to other's emotions, feelings	Little or no concern about work being done well or on time
Medium: Some attention paid to other's emotions, feelings	Moderate concern that work is being done well and on time
High: Much attention paid to other's emotions, feelings	High concern that work is being done well and on time

3. Discuss the following questions with your partner:
   a. What made me rate myself as I did?
   b. What are the advantages and disadvantages of a task orientation in nursing communication?
   c. What are the advantages and disadvantages of a person orientation in nursing communication?

Self-Disclosure

Self-disclosure means that the nurse is willing and able to talk about his or her own feelings and perceptions honestly and directly to the client. Careful use of self-disclosure can enhance a nurse–client relationship as the client views the nurse as a real person who understands his or her problems (Sundeen et al., 1989). People can be overly self-disclosing or not self-disclosing enough. An example of being overly self-disclosing is the nurse who tells everyone everything he or she is feeling all the time. Some of the nurses who work with this person will find the "nonstop" self-disclosure inappropriate or boring. On the other hand, the nurse who is totally nonself-disclosing shares few feelings or views and may well be perceived by his or her coworkers as "distant."

An additional aspect of self-disclosure is timing or appropriateness. It is possible to be self-disclosing too early in a relationship or at an inappropriate moment. Sensitivity to the client is necessary in order to determine the timing and appropriateness of self-disclosure. One way to assess your own communication style in terms of self-disclosure is with the exercise that follows.

EXERCISE IN ASSESSING SELF-DISCLOSURE

1. Rate yourself as high, medium, or low in self-disclosure when communicating with a supervisor, friend, and client about each of the following topics:
   a. Your personal life
   b. One of your personal problems
   c. Giving a big compliment
   d. Giving criticism
2. Compare your answers with those of others in the class.
3. Discuss some of the differences and similarities you find.
4. How professional do you think it is for nurses to be self-disclosing? What are the risks and payoffs?

Acceptance

Another dimension that is related to openness and self-disclosure is acceptance. Acceptance of others is a key concept in Rogers' client-centered therapy system (1951). Acceptance of both self and others is a crucial part of the therapeutic process.

What exactly is acceptance? Acceptance does not depend on one's approval of another. Some people think that acceptance means that one never gets angry or has criticism of another's actions. Needless to say, with that kind of definition, acceptance would be seen as a weakness or a trap, especially if one had to believe everything told by another person.

A working definition of acceptance is understanding that (1) what others believe or feel is their true belief or feeling, (2) others have the right to believe or feel that way, and (3) there is no need to blame others for anything they do, even if the behavior is wrong or has to be changed to protect the individual or society. The key to acceptance is allowing another the freedom to feel and think. It is only through separating the acceptance of another as a person with rights and feelings from "going along with" whatever is said or done that acceptance is a desirable and useful attribute.

How do people show that they are "accepting"? Generally, they respond to others without judging them. Thus, the nurse who can listen to a client complain about not being able to smoke in the hospital and can respond to the client's sense of frustration and (perhaps silently) disagree with the *content* of the complaints, will come across as accepting. Some of the body language the nurse might show includes head nods and a caring pat on the shoulder.

Acceptance of others is not always easy. There are few, if any, people who accept everyone all of the time. The possibility always exists that one's feelings *can* be hurt by something that is said. Frustration and disappointment can quickly turn into blame and anger. A beginning step to improve our own acceptance of others is to accept ourselves as being human, capable of mistakes and able to learn and grow from them.

Self-acceptance is like acceptance of others—we do not have to like everything we do. We may want desperately to change some things. Acceptance of ourselves involves acknowledging that, in some way, we are doing the best we can at a certain moment in time.

EXERCISE IN ACCEPTANCE OF OTHERS

1. For each of the following, rate yourself as accepting or not accepting of a supervisor, another nurse, or a client when they exhibit the following behavior of quality:

belligerence	confusion
tardiness	lying
complaining	honesty
sloppiness	criticism
affection	

2. Answer the following questions either in pairs or in a large group:
   a. Am I more accepting with some types of people than with others?
   b. Where do I get "hung up" accepting others?
   c. What happens to my communication when I am not accepting of others?
   d. Do I confuse accepting with "going along" or denying my own feelings/reactions?
   e. What are some ways I can begin to be more accepting?
   f. What are the advantages of being accepting in communicating with clients, aides, other nurses, and physicians? Are there any disadvantages?

Defensiveness

Defensiveness is a term that is usually used to describe a person's behavior in specific situations such as the nurse who responds to criticism by saying, "That's your problem." There are two overlapping meanings to the term as it is commonly used. The first meaning is that the other person is "on the defensive," being hostile, aggressive, not listening, but rather responding as if she or he were being attacked.

A second and somewhat more general definition is that the defensive person is responding by using a defense mechanism, one of several ways of defending against anxiety. Some of the major defense mechanisms include *denial,* the negation of an uncomfortable impulse or truth; *projection,* placing one's inner conflicts on others; *rationalization,* making up excuses or reasons to "cover" behavior; *reaction formation,* acting the opposite of how one feels; and *repression,* "forgetting" or putting uncomfortable thoughts or feelings out of awareness. It is important to remember that defense mechanisms are used unconsciously.

Both definitions of defensiveness have certain things in common. When persons are defensive, they are not fully able to understand the messages from others. That is, often the message is unconsciously perceived to be an attack on self-worth. The resulting response is an attempt to "save the self" but will, in all probability, mean little or be misinterpreted by another individual.

> Two nurses were working at a station when a nurse from another shift came by. One of the nurses looked up, saw her and said, "Hi! We haven't seen you for a long time." The nurse, who had been feeling guilty about being late 3 days in a row, replied, rather defensively, "Look, I work just as hard as anyone else around here!"
>
> "What's eating her?" they wondered as she left.

There are times when almost anyone acts defensively. Fatigue, hard work loads, changes in work, or personal problems can all contribute to a defensive communication style. Do any of the following areas make you feel defensive?

- Being insulted
- Being praised
- Talking about your love life
- Talking about your relationship with family members
- Having your school or professional work criticized
- Being audited by the Internal Revenue Service

EXERCISE IN SELF-DEFENSIVENESS IDENTIFICATION

1. On a piece of paper, write down three specific situations in which you have been defensive in the last 2 weeks. Include what "triggered" this reaction and what you did that was defensive.
2. Exchange lists with one other person in the class. Discuss what it is like to be "open about being defensive" with them. Share your experience in the large group or class.

One question that arises around the issue of defensiveness is how to deal with others' defensiveness. Commenting about the situation is one way to work on another's defensiveness. The following story is an example of how commenting about the situation can ease another's defensiveness.

> A nurse was assigned Mrs. Bartowski, a 76-year-old postoperative patient who was described in the nursing notes as being "abusive and angry." The nurse went over to her bed and said "Good morning, Mrs. Bartowski, how are you feeling?" "Get away from me," Mrs. B. snarled. "Mrs. Bartowski," the nurse replied, "you seem upset. Is something bothering you?" She then pulled a chair over to her bedside. Mrs. Bartowski looked at her a minute, and then tears started to form in her eyes. "Am I going to be well again?" she asked.

In this story, the key statement was the nurse's saying, "You seem upset." She was able to comment on the situation. Comments about a situation are, in technical terms, called *metacomments*. Metacomments allow the communicators to talk *about* what they see, hear, or feel the other is feeling. While metacommunicating is not a sure-fire success for another's defensiveness (after all, Mrs. Bartowski could have responded, "Nothing's bothering me, now get out of here."), it opens up a new set of options for the nurse communicator by commenting about how the other is communicating rather than simply responding to the content of what is being said.

Congruence
Another way of describing a communication style is to assess its congruence. By congruence, we mean how well the words, body language, tone of voice, and all other aspects of the communication fit together. For example, the client who bends over, grimaces, holds his hands to his stomach and says, "I

feel just wonderful," is not communicating congruently. His body language, gestures, facial expression, and probably his voice quality all say "I am feeling sick," while his words say just the opposite.

Satir (1988) has added further to the term "congruency" by noting that the message sent should be consistent with the internal feelings and beliefs of the message sender. Although some people are able to lie in a congruent way, the concept of the fit between how one feels and how one communicates is important to consider.

Does this expanded definition mean that the goal of congruency is to be perfectly honest all of the time? Fortunately, this is not the case. The question of appropriateness must also be answered in trying to be congruent. One issue in considering congruence is how to be congruent when it is *not* appropriate to share inner feelings, as in the following story:

A nurse was talking to a young mother in an outpatient clinic about care for her 12-month-old baby. The baby was with her. As the session progressed, the nurse began to notice that any time the child moved away from the mother, the mother would smile apologetically at the nurse, turn to the child, sternly say, "Stop that," and grab the child by the arm or leg. The baby eventually whimpered softly and seemed listless. The nurse became quite concerned about the interaction but knew from previous history that the woman had stopped coming into the clinic when confronted about potential child abuse by another nurse.

What would you say in this case? While there are no obvious perfect answers, several you might consider are:

- Commenting that the child seems to be healthy and active, waiting for the mother to respond to the statement, and then talking about how hard it must be to be a mother with an active child.
- Describing what the nurse sees, being very careful not to imply that the mother is wrong: "I notice that you have to tell your child to keep still often."
- Placing yourself in the other's shoes: "If I had to keep an eye on a child all the time, I'd be worn out and irritated at the end of the day."

None of the above options involve the nurse's denying his or her own feelings. (All of the options are congruent.) Metacommenting is the general strategy employed. The nurse in all three situations has a goal of attempting to help the woman verbalize parenting problems.

Instances like potential child abuse, alcoholism, and other substance abuse can be very difficult for a nurse to handle, especially when the nurse decides that direct confrontation is inappropriate and not useful for the client.

Even in less dramatic circumstances, questions can still be raised as to how to be congruent when an open statement of feelings or beliefs is too costly, for example, in a situation where you could lose your job. One guiding concept is: given the range of choices for communicating (including doing nothing!), what can you do that does not violate your feelings, beliefs, or standards?

COMMUNICATION STYLES: SATIR'S CATEGORIES

Another way of looking at communication styles is to categorize them, that is, to imagine common patterns in the way we communicate. Several authors have devised methods of categorizing communication styles. One that the authors of this book have found to be quite useful in understanding nursing communication is the system devised by Virginia Satir. We recommend her books, *The New Peoplemaking* (1988) and *Making Contact* (1976), to those readers who are interested in finding out more about communication styles. The explanation that follows is a shortened version of the Satir communication model with specific examples related to nursing.

There are two concepts that are important to understand before examining Satir's communication styles. They are the concepts of *self-worth* and *stress*.

Self-Worth

In Satir's system, self-worth is a major influence on all communication. Self-worth is the positive value we place on ourselves as individuals. It can be our greatest asset in human interactions. An understanding of one's own self-worth is essential in being able to communicate effectively with others. This is true for nursing as well as other professions.

We depend to a large extent on the reactions of others to determine who we really are. These reactions provide a reflection for us to view ourselves. All of us would like to have a positive regard for ourselves, to view ourselves as mature people. At the same time, we frequently depend on the reactions of others to determine who we really are. Self-worth can get in the way of praise, blame, criticism, and fairly routine exchanges, even though message senders are not evaluating or judging the other person; only their behavior. It is easy for nurses in leadership roles to forget how easily self-worth becomes involved in evaluations of another's work or in normal informational exchanges. Students have difficulty separating self-worth from their performance as nurses. We all equate high levels of performance with self-worth. Self-worth can also interfere with how we perceive the actions of others. This is shown in the following example:

Two nurses were comparing notes about a head nurse. The first one said, "She's great. She takes time to show me how to do procedures I don't understand and makes sure I do things right." The second looked at her with surprise on his face. "What do you mean?" he retorted. "She's always telling me what to do. She tries to control everything. She must think we're pretty stupid."

It is possible that the second nurse is allowing his feelings of "low" self-worth to influence his perception of the head nurse's motives. In fact, the head nurse may have been trying to help him. However, his lowered self-image contributes not only to his dislike for himself, but to thinking that the head nurse, who may have been acting appropriately, disliked him as well.

Sometimes we form unconscious links between our degree of self-worth and certain feelings. That is, self-worth is often low because of a self-inflicted rule that says, "I am a bad person because I feel angry, sad, incompetent, crazy, stupid, upset, or anything else." For example, nurses might feel low self-worth if they are "mad" at a client or if they cannot solve another client's problem. These two examples represent instances of feeling low self-worth because of a feeling (anger) or a rule (only feeling self-worth when a client's problems are solved). There is no reason that self-worth has to be lowered due to a feeling or to failing in a task. In fact, keeping one's sense of high self-worth can help us in changing undesired behavior. "Self-assessment," in which one uncovers the unconscious links between self-worth and feelings or behavior, is one important step towards the growth of the adult individual, as well as promoting understanding.

Stress

In Satir's system, stress, which is closely related to self-worth, is felt whenever self-worth is threatened. This means that we tend to feel stress whenever we unconsciously link feelings or the behavior or words of others with a lowering of our own sense of self-worth. The link may be uncalled for, but it is made. Stress is felt when self-worth is endangered.

People respond to stress in many ways. Consider the following situation:

Kim (nurse 1) was talking to her friend John (nurse 2) about a "problem client" with whom she had had no success in terms of adherence to medical orders. The client, who was supposed to be staying in bed, was always getting up and walking around. "I finally had someone else talk to him," she stated. "Why didn't you confront him?" John asked.

At this point, Kim, if she interprets the question (unconsciously or consciously) as an attack on her self-worth, may respond in one of the following defensive ways:

Blaming: That's none of your business. You always question me!
Placating: You're right. I was wrong, it was my fault. I'm so sorry I did my job badly.

Superreasonable: Studies have shown that in 75 percent of cases similar to these, a different nurse has more success. Thus, I decided to utilize the research data in coming to the problem solution.

Irrelevant: He wasn't good-looking enough to be worth the trouble.

There is also the possibility that Kim could respond congruently:

Congruent: I decided to let someone else try. I was having no success and felt frustrated.

The first four responses represent noncongruent responses. That is, they are as much responses to internal stress as they are to the question. Furthermore, they are not particularly useful in helping nurses talk about how they feel *or* how they feel about what their feelings are (metacommenting about self-worth). The fifth response, the congruent response, was one in which feelings were accurately verbalized, and self-worth was separated from behavior. In this way, John's question was treated as an inquiry rather than as an attack and the question that was asked was answered.

This simple scenario points out the complexity of any communication. The major aspects are:

1. Nurse 1's behavior
2. Nurse 1's feelings about what was done
3. Nurse 1's self-worth about what was done
4. Nurse 2's question
5. Nurse 2's feelings or reactions to nurse 1 at that moment in time
6. Nurse 2's feelings of self-worth at that moment in time
7. Nurse 1's response to nurse 2's question
8. Nurse 1's feelings upon hearing the question
9. Nurse 1's feelings of self-worth about her own feelings from hearing the question

For the sake of presentation, it was assumed that nurse 2's comment was congruent and not presented in a stressful manner. Imagine the potential confusion, miscommunication, and hurt feelings that might have ensued if both nurses had their self-worth involved where it did not belong!

The nine actions in the example just presented can be grouped into three general aspects of a communication: the self, the other, and the context.

Satir represents them as shown in Figure 3–1. *Self* refers to one's feelings, perception, and self-worth in a given communication. *Other* refers to the other person's feelings, perceptions, and self-worth in the communication. *Context* refers to both the context in which the communication takes place and the specific content of the communication.

One of the major attributes of noncongruent communication styles is that each partner ignores at least one aspect of the self–other–context configuration. Another disadvantage of noncongruent styles is that they do not successfully alleviate stress. They do not allow metacommenting, talking

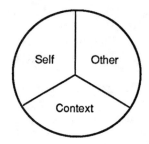

Figure 3–1. The three general aspects of communication according to Satir's model.

about feelings of what is going on. They are often misunderstood and are not a free choice as a response. When people act in a noncongruent way (blaming, placating, being superreasonable or irrelevant), they are not consciously choosing that response category. They are simply trying (unsuccessfully) to protect their self-worth; to say, "I count; I am OK."

Each of the noncongruent response styles has its own characteristics, physical postures (body language), language uses, and effects on others. By reading about and practicing the noncongruent responses, we can begin to identify them in our own nursing communication, as well as begin to discover them in others. This, in turn, should help us become more congruent and effective nurse communicators.

Blaming

The first response Kim gave to John in the earlier example was, "That's none of your business. You always question me." In this response, while Kim is responding to her own needs and the content of John's question, she is not taking John's feelings into account. At the same time, John is given responsibility for the blamer's behavior ("*you* always question me"). A diagram of the blaming response is represented in Figure 3–2. When someone blames, while he or she defends the self and pays attention to the issues, the other person is attacked. The blamer frequently disagrees.

The language used in blaming includes the frequent occurrence of the following words and phrases:

you always	never
should	you made me
no	it's your fault

These words are usually said in a hostile manner, although we all know some subtle blamers who seem to "make" us feel guilty, depressed, or put down even though they do not seem to be very hostile.

The body language of the blamer is most easily characterized by the "blaming finger." There is tremendous power in finger pointing. One can most readily observe the "blaming finger" in supermarkets. Adults are able to immobilize a child at 30 paces without speaking a word.

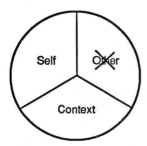

Figure 3–2. Representation of the blamer's denial of the aspect of the "other."

Other parts of the body language of blaming include tight arm and neck muscles, clenching the teeth, and tightening of facial muscles. A caricature of the blamer would be a person standing, one foot in front of the other, leaning forward, and glaring, with one hand on the hip, and the other hand extended and pointing at the person with whom the blamer is "communicating."

People respond to blame in many ways. What usually happens is that people who are blamed feel guilty, hurt, angry, put down, and occasionally blame in return. Usually all that is seen is the blaming finger, not the scared self-worth hiding behind it. One thing is certain; blaming does not foster effective communication. The following exercise is designed to have you *consciously* practice blame.

EXERCISE 1 IN BLAMING

1. Pair up. One partner will be *A*, the other *B*.
2. *A* puts the following statements into blaming terms by tone of voice, gestures, or changing the words. *B* listens and gives feedback, telling *A* if *A* is a "successful" blamer. You may be dramatic as you do this.

   STATEMENTS
   a. I disagree with you.
   b. Do you like me?
   c. What is your problem?
   d. Did you sleep well?
   e. What time is it?
3. Then, *B* will practice blaming *A* by changing the following statements into blaming statements. *A* listens. Again, *B* can be dramatic.
   a. You need to take your medicine.
   b. How are you today?
   c. Can you try harder?
   d. You will be well in a week.
   e. You have a lot of visitors.

EXERCISE 2 IN BLAMING

1. Pair up. One partner will be *A*, the other *B*.
2. *A* will say the following statements two ways; first in a caring way and then in as blaming a manner as possible without changing the words. *B* listens and asks *A* to do it again if *A* does not blame well.
   a. You do not look well.
   b. What's the matter with you?
   c. Please sit up.
   d. Put out your tongue.
   e. Show me the medicine you have.
3. Switch roles. *B* will then say the following statements two ways; first in a caring manner, then in a blaming manner. (*A* listens and makes *B* do it again if *B* does not blame well.)
   a. Your gown is on backwards.
   b. Do you have a problem?
   c. I'm very busy now.
   d. Is your daughter home?
   e. Did Mr. Jones die?
4. Discuss the subtle ways in which blame can be added to statements.
5. Discuss how a client might feel blamed when being given instructions on procedures.

Placating

The second response Kim gave in the situation described earlier was: "You're right. I was wrong. It was my fault. I'm so sorry I do my job badly." In this instance, Kim is respecting John's view but is not respecting herself as a person. She "puts herself down," assumes total responsibility for everything, and is overly apologetic. (It *is* possible to apologize without placating.) Figure 3–3 presents a diagram of the placator's communication. Similar to the blamer's ignoring the feelings of the other and yet putting responsibility on oneself, the placater ignores his or her own feelings yet takes responsibility for everyone else. ("It's my fault, I made you do it.") What a way to communicate! Yet, again, the placater is trying (unsuccessfully) to say, "I count, I'm OK."

The language of the placater is agreement. A placater will make peace at any cost, appease others, and agree to conflicting opinions. In other words, a placater tries to be nice no matter what.

When we placate we are acting as if the only way to be "OK" is to agree. How many times have we agreed to things we did not want to do just to be nice? How many clients nod their heads yes in agreement as if they understand instructions but really do not? In the same manner that the blamer disagrees, the placater automatically agrees with everyone.

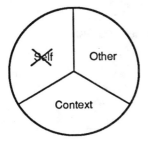

Figure 3–3. Representation of the placater's denial of the aspect of the "self."

Phrases and words commonly used to placate include:

Yes	You are right
I made you do it	I don't deserve you
I'm so sorry	I apologize
It's my fault	I'm wrong
I'm to blame	I should do better

These words can, of course, be used without placating; but with the proper intonation, physical gestures, and body language, they can give a strong placating impression.

The body language of the placater is that of supplication. Wrung hands, held up as if they were pleading, the head held low, eyes lifted slightly, as if asking for forgiveness, the shoulders rounded, somewhat slouched, the body hunched over as if saying, "I'm no good," one leg is in front of the other, perhaps in a caricature sense, being on one knee—all are placating gestures. Ordinary responses to placaters are anger, pity, slight disgust, and "tuning out." The big problem with placaters is that one never knows how they feel, what they think, or what they really want because they are too busy trying to appease.

The next two exercises are designed to give you practice placating. The more you can consciously placate, the more you will be aware of yourself unintentionally placating in other situations.

EXERCISE 1 IN PLACATING

1. Pair up. One partner will be *A*, the other *B*.
2. *A* will put the following statements into placating terms. *B* listens and gives feedback. A can be dramatic as she or he translates the statements.
   a. I need more help with my clients.
   b. Doctor, can you see Mr. Jones?
   c. Where is the client's chart?
   d. Have you seen a doctor recently?
   e. Does your child eat a balanced diet?

3. *B* will then translate the following nursing communication into placating statements. Be dramatic. *A* will provide feedback.
   a. What is Mr. Smith's address?
   b. Do you want a back rub?
   c. Doctor, what's the diagnosis?
   d. I need some help in here immediately!
   e. I'm here to help with discharge planning.

EXERCISE 2 IN PLACATING

1. *A* will say each of the following statements two ways, first in an ordinary conversational tone, then placating. Be dramatic. (*B* listens and makes *A* repeat if *A* does not placate well).
   a. I'm sorry I had to wake you.
   b. Good morning, I'm the V.N.A. nurse.
   c. Doctor, can I help you?
   d. I need to ambulate the client.
   e. Where is the client who is going to surgery?
2. *B* will then do the same exercise with the following statements:
   a. Doctor, did you see Mrs. Bova?
   b. Has anyone seen Dr. Cartone?
   c. I didn't mean to disturb you.
   d. I was wrong to call you in for this.
   e. I'll be through with you in a minute.
3. Discuss how clients might react to a nurse who placates.

Being Superreasonable

The third response Kim made was to be superreasonable: "Studies have shown that in 75 percent of cases similar to these, a different nurse has more success. Thus, I decided to use research data in coming to the problem solution." When people are being superreasonable, they appear to be quite intelligent but are, in fact, using their minds to avoid their feelings. What comes out sounds rational but is not truly creative thought. No attention is paid to the feelings of self or other. Thus, a diagram of the three aspects for a superreasonable communication would be represented by Figure 3–4. All that matters is the content. Feelings are to be avoided at all cost.

There are times when it is quite appropriate to communicate only content. Giving data about a client at report is one example. The difference between useful factualness and superreasonableness lies in how the brain is being used. Does what is being said involve ignoring relevant feelings or beliefs? If so, the communicator is being superreasonable.

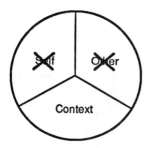

Figure 3–4. Representation of the denial of the aspects of both "self" and "other" in being superreasonable.

The language of superreasonable is impersonal. Facts are substituted for "I believe" or "I feel." There is a frequent use of categorical statements such as "It is clear that" or "It is true that." Other phrases commonly used when people are being superreasonable include:

- Let the facts speak for themselves
- It said in the paper (book, article)
- There is no logical reason
- There is every logical reason
- Let's be rational about this

The body language of the superreasonable person is rigid and upright. There is no eye contact, since a superreasonable person is interested only in the facts. The caricatured superreasonable person is standing ramrod straight, arms at the side, looking off into the distance. The tone of voice is a monotone, and his or her words are spoken as if they came from a computer printout.

It is very difficult to respond with compassion to a person who is being superreasonable. Some common responses people have to superreasonableness include feeling they do not exist, feeling hurt, frustration, or even becoming superreasonable in return. The following exercises will give you practice in experiencing and identifying superreasonableness.

EXERCISE 1 IN SUPERREASONABLENESS

1. Pair up. One partner will be *A*, the other *B*.
2. *A* will "translate" the following set of statements into superreasonable communication. For example, a superreasonable "translation" of "Do not upset the client" is "Are you aware of the fact that the way you are communicating has been shown to elevate clients' blood pressures?" *B* listens and has *A* do it again if *A* is not superreasonable.
   a. Do not upset the client.
   b. It's time for the report.

c. This client needs a bath.
d. That temperature is very high.
e. You really seem depressed.
3. Now switch roles. *B* translates the following statements into super-reasonable communication:
a. I am not sure the medication is correct.
b. There must be an explanation for this.
c. Have you been following your regimen?
d. Your father is in room 29.
e. Is everything OK?

EXERCISE 2 IN SUPERREASONABLENESS

1. Pair up. One partner will be *A*, the other *B*.
2. *A* will repeat each of the following sentences in two ways: first in a conversational and caring manner, then in a superreasonable manner. *B* will listen and have *A* do it again if *A* is not superreasonable enough. (Hint to *A*: be sure to make no eye contact when you are being superreasonable. Staring above *B*'s head is an excellent tactic.)
a. Did you eat all of your meal?
b. You look like you are in pain.
c. Is the tourniquet too tight?
d. Children need attention from their parents.
e. I want you to know the side effects of your medicine.
3. *B* will then repeat each of the following statements in the same way, first in a caring manner, then superreasonably. *A* will listen and have *B* repeat any that are not done in a superreasonable manner.
a. You will go to surgery tomorrow.
b. Your husband is better today.
c. I need to talk to you about a personal matter.
d. Did someone forget to replace the chart?
e. We need another nurse on this floor.
4. Discuss how clients might react to a nurse who is being superreasonable.

Irrelevance

The fourth response Kim gave was to be irrelevant: "He wasn't good-looking enough for me to bother." Irrelevancy is the fine art of avoiding the issue, ignoring your own feelings, and ignoring the feelings of others. The irrelevant response communication diagram is seen in Figure 3–5.

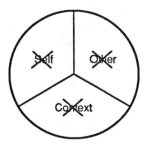

Figure 3–5. Representation of the denial of all aspects of appropriate communication in being irrelevant.

Irrelevant behavior is distracting, occasionally amusing, and hard to follow. There may be many words spoken, but few are to the point. Some common phrases used in irrelevant communication include:

- Wait a minute, let me tell you about . . .
- That reminds me of the one about . . .
- By the way (followed by a change of topic)

The key to irrelevancy is not the specific words used, but the manner in which they are used to change the subject and avoid alluding to feelings.

The body language of the person using an irrelevant response is that of motion and distraction. He or she is "all over the place" (except for being centered on the matter at hand).

Others respond to irrelevance by being confused, impatient, anxious, and occasionally angry. Clearly, irrelevance does not make communication any better.

At the same time, levity, humor, and perspective can be beneficial in a work setting. Irrelevancy can be distinguished from these attributes in that self, other, and context are ignored, and the irrelevancy is inappropriate for the situation.

The following exercise will help you practice being irrelevant.

EXERCISE 1 IN IRRELEVANCY

1. Pair up. One partner will be *A*, the other *B*.
2. *A* will then translate the following statements into irrelevant statements. For example, an irrelevant version of "I need to give you your shot now" is "I notice that you had a visitor." *B*'s job is to listen and have *A* make sure *A* is irrelevant.
   a. I need to give you your shot now.
   b. I feel badly about Mrs. Jones' progress.
   c. Doctor, the client has been waiting 1 hour.
   d. I am very confused about Mrs. Castillo's tumor.
   e. We have to pass out meds more carefully.

3. Switch so *B* translates the following statements into irrelevant statements. *A*'s job is to listen and have *B* try again if he or she is not irrelevant.
   a. The kardex is missing.
   b. Does Mr. Rivera have an internist?
   c. What is this client's blood pressure?
   d. This child's cast is cracked.
   e. How many cigarettes do you smoke a day?

EXERCISE 2 IN IRRELEVANCY

1. Pair up. One partner will be *A*, the other *B*.
2. *A* will then say each of the following in an irrelevant manner. *B* listens and makes *A* do any that are not irrelevant over again (hint: use a lot of body distraction).
   a. I have to talk to you, doctor, about this.
   b. Mrs. Buffard, are you warm enough?
   c. Your gown is in the closet.
   d. Whose dentures are these?
   e. Have you seen Joseph?
3. Switch so that *B* says the same statements in an irrelevant, but different, manner than *A* did. Discuss variations in how one can be irrelevant.
4. Discuss the impact of being irrelevant on other nurses and clients.

Congruence

There is a fifth choice responding to stress. This choice is to be congruent; that is, the words and actions in a communication fit the inner experience of self and are appropriate to the context. A congruent response takes the other person's feelings into account and does not allow feelings of "low" self-worth to influence the communication process. A congruent response is healthy, as opposed to the other four responses—which are not. By healthy, it is meant that tension is decreased and self-worth is at a high level.

There are no magical congruent phrases (phrases that are *always* congruent) or magical congruent postures; no one stance of a person is necessarily congruent in all situations. However, certain phrases and statements from the four noncongruent categories can be restated in a more congruent manner. That is, they can be restated differently, taking away implied blame, placation, superreasonableness, and irrelevance. Generally, the "translation" includes using the word "I" for ownership of feelings of belief ("I think that ... ," "It is my feeling that . . .") or a lessening of categorical phrases ("always," "should," "never") to a more accurate statement of reality ("for now," "at this moment").

Blame: Mr. Jones, why are you being stupid? You should never leave the bed by yourself!!!

Congruent: Mr. Jones, you are not supposed to leave your bed without help according to the doctor. Please call me the next time you have to get up.

Blame: I don't care if you're the head nurse, don't you ever talk to me like that!

Congruent: I feel you are being hard on me.

Placate: I'm so sorry to bother you, Dr. Barker, but . . . it's my fault I know . . . Mrs. Bailey is complaining of pain, I'm sorry.

Congruent: Dr. Barker, Mrs. Bailey is complaining of pain.

Superreasonable: Ninety-eight percent of all post-op patients have variable control over their locomotion and gaint, Mr. Peterson.

Congruent: It may take you some time to walk well after that operation.

Irrelevant: Hello Jonesy, what's new? Did you have trouble parking? (Jonesy is 10 minutes late for her shift.)

Congruent: You were 10 minutes late. I'd like you to be on time.

A tendency to blame, when transformed by adding high self-worth and respect for others, can become an assertive request. Placating, when transformed by adding high self-worth and self-respect, can become care for others. Superreasonableness, when transformed by adding high self-worth and respect for one's own and others' feelings, can become creative intelligence. Irrelevancy, when transformed by adding high self-worth and respect for self, respect for others as well as respect for context, becomes humor and a sense of perspective. These transformations are summarized in Table 3–1.

TABLE 3–1. CONGRUENT RESPONSES

Response		Missing Pieces		Congruent Transformation
Blame	+	Respect for other's feelings	=	Assertion
Placating	+	Self-respect	=	Care, concern
Superreasonableness	+	Respect for other's feelings + respect for own feelings	=	Intelligence
Irrelevance	+	Respect for self + respect for others + respect for the context	=	Humor, perspective, ability to make connections

CONCLUSION

All persons have unique and varying styles of communication. Six of these styles, as well as related exercises, have been presented in this chapter to enable nurses to assess their own communication styles and those of clients more accurately.

A knowledge of Satir's communication framework and its relation to the concepts of self-worth and stress provide a foundation for understanding defensive behavior. Defensive behavior occurs when one's self-worth is threatened or one feels under stress. Four patterns of defensive behavior—blaming, placating, superreasonableness, and irrelevancy are usually unhealthy responses. A fifth pattern, congruence, is a healthy response. There are some nursing situations and role relationships in which nurses might find themselves using "noncongruent" or defensive behaviors, fully aware of their decision to do so. For example, if nurses needed help in a medical emergency, they might yell or "blame." What has been emphasized in this chapter is that nurse communicators can make choices, based on the situational needs, rather than responding from a position of low self-worth.

REFERENCES

Blake, R. R., Mouton, J. S., & Tapper, M. *Grid approaches for managerial leadership in nursing.* St. Louis: C. V. Mosby Co., 1981.

Murray, B., & Zentner, J. P. *Nursing assessment and health promotion strategies through the life span* (4th ed.). Norwalk, Conn.: Appleton & Lange, 1989.

Rogers, C. *Client centered therapy.* Boston: Houghton Mifflin, 1951.

Satir, V. *Making contact.* Millbrae, Calif.: Celestial Arts, 1976.

Satir, V. *The new peoplemaking.* Palo Alto, Calif.: Science and Behavior Books, 1988.

Sundeen, S. J., Stuart, G. W., Rankin, E. A., & Cohen, S. A. *Nurse–client interaction* (4th ed.). St. Louis: C. V. Mosby Co., 1989.

4 Therapeutic Use of Self, Trust, and Empathy

BEHAVIORAL OBJECTIVES

By reading this chapter and participating in the exercises, students will be able to:

1. Identify three concepts that promote helping relationships: therapeutic use of self, development of a sense of trust, and the use of empathy
2. Describe four verbal skills relating to trust and empathy: the use of "I" statements, reflection, sharing feelings, and verbal reassurance
3. Discuss four nonverbal skills relating to trust and empathy: nonverbal reassurance, attending to the client, active listening, and the use of silence

This chapter focuses on three general concepts: therapeutic use of self, trust, and empathy. These concepts contain both concrete (high visibility) and abstract (low visibility) elements. They are complex and do not necessarily occur in every nurse–client relationship. Clients will not automatically trust nurses nor will nurses automatically use an empathic approach when interacting with clients. Some clients will be more amenable to developing a sense of trust, however, and, similarly, some nurses will find it easy to develop a therapeutic approach to clients.

THERAPEUTIC USE OF SELF

Most nurses want to help people; that is one of the major reasons they elected to enter the field of nursing. Helping is a natural occurrence in everyday life. We find ourselves helping others many times during the course of a day; responding to the requests of others or assisting in small tasks. These requests or tasks have a goal; they tend to solve a problem. They also foster a relationship between two people—a relationship that is essentially a partnership. Each partner gives and receives in the relationship in nearly equal proportions.

A helping relationship in a nurse–client interaction is different. Although the goal, that of problem solving, is the same, one person (the nurse) is giving more than the other (the client). The nurse or helper is providing conditions for the client or helpee to meet his or her needs (Brammer, 1988). In all helping relationships, you bring the totality of your experiences—your values, feelings, and attitudes into the communication; however, the basic objectives of these two interactions differ. You usually talk to your friend to socialize, to get to know each other better, to obtain or share information. While you may talk to clients for these same reasons, you also talk to them to establish trusting relationships, to allow for expression of feelings, or to help them to realize personal goals that will help them to regain their independence.

The nurse's role in such helping relationships is a therapeutic role, that is, the nurse interacts with the client for the expressed purpose of benefiting the client. The use of self in a therapeutic way in which the client's needs are the central focus characterizes communication interactions. The nurse guides, directs, and structures the communication interactions in such a way that the client is able to verbalize feelings. Rogers (1961) defines a helping relationship as one that "intentionally promotes growth and development, improved functioning and improved coping with life of the other."

Therapeutic use of self *does not* have to be done dramatically. Many normal nursing functions can be performed in a therapeutic manner. For example, many clients recovering from a stroke or a long bed rest have difficulty walking in part due to low confidence in their physical powers. When the nurse takes such a client's arm and walks with him or her, the nurse is able to act as a prosthesis or extension of the person. But there is something more. There is kinesthetic communication. It is as if the confidence and stability of one person (the nurse) passes to the other (the client), and the client is able to walk with confidence and can assume a more normal gait. Although this is an example of the nurse extending herself or himself therapeutically to fulfill a client's physical need, psychological needs are fulfilled in much the same manner.

The following two exercises are designed to help you begin to conceptualize how to use yourself therapeutically in nursing activities. Keep in mind that the therapeutic use of self is a complicated skill that can require months or even years of training.

EXERCISE 1 IN THERAPEUTIC USE OF SELF

In the large group, discuss each of the following procedures in *two* ways; first, in terms of *how* to perform the nursing procedure; second, how to utilize "therapeutic use of self" while performing the procedure.

1. Taking a blood pressure
2. Bathing a client
3. Administering medication
4. Discussing medication compliance with a client
5. Home safety assessment

EXERCISE 2 IN THERAPEUTIC USE OF SELF

1. Pair up. One partner will be *A*, the other *B*. *A* is to think of a situation or problem that is of real concern and one that *A* would like to change.
2. *A* shares the problem with *B*. Be brief and specific, but at the same time, share some of the reasons for your concern. *B*'s task is to guide the interaction in such a way that *A* is able to focus on the concern. *B* should resist the temptation to talk about him- or herself.
3. Switch roles and repeat steps 2–4.
4. Discuss the interactions, asking yourself if you were able to demonstrate the "therapeutic use of self."

DEVELOPMENT OF A SENSE OF TRUST

The ability to use oneself therapeutically in a nursing situation is directly related to the client's level of trust. Trust is central to a therapeutic nurse–client relationship. Without a sense of trust, the interaction is superficial, with little personal involvement of either the client or the nurse.

What exactly is trust and how is it communicated? Trust is relying on someone without question. It is developed through communication that is forthright and honest. Clients trust nurses who can demonstrate skill and experience. Thus, trust is related to confidence, dependability, and credibility in a relationship.

Trust is also related to the goals and aims of the nurse; are these goals congruent with the goals of the client? If so, then both client and nurse cooperate to achieve these goals in an atmosphere of trust.

It usually takes an extended period of time for persons to develop a sense of trust with each other. In nursing interactions one hears the term "levels of trust," that is, the development of trust progresses through a series of sequential phases: the orientation phase, the working phase, and the termination phase (Sundeen et al., 1989). Although the transition from one phase to another is gradual and each phase varies in length of time, there are characteristics which can be attributed to each, whether it be in the development of trust or in the development of the nurse–client relationship itself.

Phase I—Orientation Phase

This period is characterized by the superficial or beginning level of the relationship, and it can be marked by uncertainty and exploration. Both nurse and client are beginning to clarify their respective roles through the mutual provision of such information as name, how, when, how long and how often, and purpose of the interaction. There is a mutual "feeling out" of what is expected. In this initial phase, nursing goals and their related outcomes are set. These goals can be either formal or informal, formal implying that a contract has been written.

The formation of trust begins in the orientation phase of the nurse–client relationship and can be impeded by either the nurse or client. Nurses who have the ability to trust *usually* will enable clients to develop a sense of trust. It is important for nurses to be able to disclose themselves in order to let clients know them. To disclose in a meaningful way, nurses must take the risk that clients will reject them. The willingness to risk rejection is part of the trust relationship. On the other hand, clients who have had negative interpersonal experiences in the past with nurses in relation to emotional and physical health care outcomes can have difficulty in developing trust. These clients are less able to take risks until they have first tested the other person in the interaction. Finally, in developing trust with clients, nurses have an advantage. They know more about the client than the client knows about them. They have read the client's chart, heard reports about the client, know the client's age and diagnosis, and so forth.

Phase II—Working Phase

In the second phase of trust development, the boundaries of the relationship are more flexible, as the stereotypic roles of "nurse" and "client" are shed. The nurse is no longer a symbol in a uniform, but a person; the client becomes a person with feelings. Both the nurse and client are willing to share feelings and discuss in greater detail those concerns touched upon in the orientation phase. They are now comfortable with an increasing awareness of self as well as their own goals and motivations, and they share this awareness with each other. The client has moved from an external to an internal frame of reference, and inner concerns central to the client (not the nurse) become the focus of the interaction. Confidentiality is established. The nurse may self-disclose, but only in the service of therapeutically attending to the client.

> Client: Nobody cares what happens to me.
> Nurse: I feel the same way sometimes. It is not easy to face an operation.

Phase III—Termination

This phase occurs when encounters between the nurse and client are ending. It can begin on first contact when the nurse states the relationship will end (Brill & Kilts, 1986). A sudden and unannounced departure, especially when there has been a strong personal investment, can leave the client in a state of mistrust and cause separation anxiety. This makes it all the more difficult to develop a sense of trust in future relationships.

Student nurses, by virtue of their short contact with clients, often fall prey to a sense of mistrust on the part of the client because they fail to inform clients when they will terminate the relationship. Clients, as much as they love students, often find it difficult to share feelings because of the temporary nature of the nurse–client interaction. When nurses interact with clients on an intermittent basis, such as in an ambulatory care clinic, clients are usually not seen by the same nurse during each subsequent visit. Such follow-up nursing care, such as dietary or weight changes, or compliance to medical regimens, is not reinforced by the same nurse. The establishment of a trusting relationship between nurse and client is followed by an abrupt termination of the relationship. This not only creates stress for the nursing staff but mandates accurate and comprehensive documentation on clients' medical records. A direct acknowledgement by the nurse of both the shortness of the contact and feelings about it are beneficial in preventing a sense of loss and in developing a sense of trust in these circumstances.

USE OF EMPATHY

Empathy is an essential element of the interpersonal process and when communicated, forms the basis for a helping relationship between nurse and client. Empathy implies the ability to put one's self in the other person's shoes—to feel as well as to graph intellectually the other person's plight (Albert & Wittenberg, 1986). Empathy is defined as "a psychological *process*

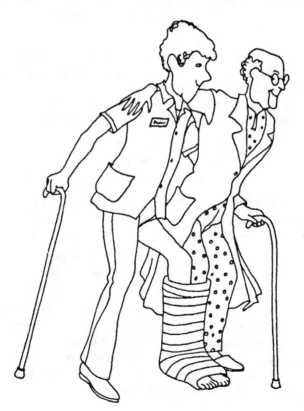

of a nurse feeling into a client's thinking; sensing, comprehending, and sharing his/her internal frame of reference" (Janzen, 1984, p. 3). Empathic nurses enter into the lives of their clients and respond in the client's language and terms, using the same feeling tone of voice: sad if the client is sad or fearful if the client is fearful. Empathic nurses are able to achieve a deeper appreciation and understanding of the client as a unique individual, and clients feel a greater sense of reassurance and acceptance. This process has three components: the empathic state of the nurse, the communication of empathy from nurse to client, and the perception of a nurse's empathic state by the client. Empathy, therefore, involves both the nurse's sensitivity to the client's current feelings as well as the nurse's verbal facility to communicate this understanding in a language attuned to the client's current feelings.

One way to conceptualize empathy is to look at a three-dimensional model presented for nurses by Schwartz et al. (1983). The model includes three discrete approaches to empathy.

1.   *The predictive approach:* the ability to accurately predict the thoughts and feelings of others, that is, take on their role, even if the attitudes are different from one's own.

     EXAMPLE: I am empathic if I can take on your role and accurately know how you think and feel even if you are very different from me.

2.   *The achieved approach:* an interactive client-centered approach. The thoughts and feelings of the other, while not becoming yours, need to be perceived by the other as being understood. Instead of focusing on accurate understanding (as in the predictive approach), here the focus is on whether the other person feels understood.

     EXAMPLE: I am empathic if you think I understand you, that is, you perceive me as understanding you. I have achieved empathy because you believe that I understand.

3.   *The behavioral approach:* this approach is not an accurate understanding of the source or perceived understanding by the receiver, but focuses on behaviors which promote understanding.

     EXAMPLE: I am empathic if I can make appropriate statements in response to you. This would include responses in all channels.

Empathy differs from sympathy. The sympathetic nurse is subjective, as opposed to the empathic nurse who maintains a sense of objectivity. The sympathetic nurse offers condolence and pity, whereas the empathic nurse offers support and understanding. A skilled nurse communicator empathizes rather than sympathizes. Fortunately, it is not necessary to totally experience the client's feelings in order to be helpful. Nurses can help if they *understand* how the other person feels. That is what is meant by empathy (Gazda, Childers, & Walters, 1982). The difference between empathy and sympathy is shown in the following example:

> A nurse's assignment included Jimmy, an 8-year-old boy who had been hospitalized with leukemia for several months. Jimmy's mother was often present when the nurse gave care. The mother had adapted to Jimmy's illness and wanted to have as much contact as possible with her son.
>   The nurse was responding to the situation with sympathy. She felt very sorry for Jimmy and was often on the verge of tears while working with him. She also found herself close to tears when the mother was present. The nurse felt that neither mother nor child would understand her tears, so she would frequently leave the room. The nurse did not include the mother in bathing her son or in other appropriate procedures.

By sympathizing with Jimmy, the nurse became an obstacle to empathic communication rather than a facilitator of therapeutic nursing care. With an empathic approach, the nurse could have included the mother in the care, and the nurse could have shared tears with the family. Note that crying is not necessarily unprofessional, as long as it fits the context and the relationship between the nurse and others. The idea of "sharing tears with" (an empathic approach) is quite different from "shedding tears for" (a sympathetic approach).

Numerous references have been made to the empathic process in the nursing literature. This leads one to ask why empathy is so important to nursing. High empathic nurses are able to establish an accurate understanding of the client from the client's frame of reference; they also establish rapport by keeping channels open for clients to express feelings and concerns. The use of empathy has a direct relationship to client improvement, for example, regardless of the specific diagnosis or prognosis, it increases one's ability to cope with a terminal illness and/or cancer (DiMatteo & Friedman, 1982).

Nurses have attempted in the past to articulate the empathic process through measurement with empathy rating scales, for example, the Barrett-Lennard Relationship Inventory (1962), the Truax Accurate Empathy Scale (1961, 1963), and Carkhuff's Empathy Scales (1969). These instruments confirm the lack of agreement among researchers on the theoretical and operational definitions of empathy. Janzen (1984) conducted a thorough review of the literature and found that established empathy rating scales did not correlate with each other. She concluded that there is either a problem with the definition of empathy or with the standardized instruments being used to measure empathy in nursing.

Research conducted by nurses using rehearsal and various modeling techniques has addressed the issue of *how* nurses' empathy is communicated to clients. They have concluded there is little relationship between empathy and communication, particularly in terms of verbal communication. This in turn suggests that an empathic state is not transmitted by words; rather nonverbal communication plays a powerful role (Janzen, 1984). Nonverbal communication is a condition of perceived empathy and as such can be taught by emphasizing the use of specific observable behaviors, such as physical proximity, forward lean, eye contact, shoulder orientation to the helpee, and arm openness.

VERBAL SKILLS RELATING TO TRUST AND EMPATHY

Four verbal skills that nurses can learn to use in order to increase the likelihood of developing an atmosphere of trust and empathy through the therapeutic use of self are the use of "I" statements, reflection, sharing feelings, and verbal reassurance.

"I" Statements

The use of the word "I" is an assertive behavior that can be used by nurses as a way of helping clients own their own feelings (Palmer & Deck, 1987). The general view behind this is that as an individual says "I feel" or "I believe" (as opposed to "you make me feel" or "the truth is"), he or she will make a more accurate statement and come across in a less dogmatic or pedantic fashion.

The first issue is when to use "I." Obviously, there are times when "I" is inappropriate. For example, if it's time for a client's bath, you would say something like "It's time for your bath, Mr. Jones" or possibly "I see it's time for your bath." The common use of the word "we" to mean "you" is *not* recommended. In the example above, saying "It's time for our bath" is incorrect. Only one person is being bathed, and that is the client. The inappropriate use of the word "we" is at best confusing and at worst condescending.

So the question still remains as to when do you, the nurse, use "I"? The following contexts serve as a partial list. Can you think of any others?

- Requesting information (I would like you to ...)
- Asking the client to comply (I would like you to ...)
- Giving your opinion (I think that ...)
- Discussing feelings (I hear you saying ...)
- Giving suggestions (I think you could ...)

As is the case with any technique, "I" statements can also be misused. For example, it is possible to communicate defensively with an "I" statement, such as "I feel so sorry, it's all my fault, doctor" (placating) or "I hate you, I won't do it!!!" (blaming). It is also possible to dominate a conversation or overdo "I" statements. If every sentence a nurse says begins with "I think," others will start to tune out the nurse's communication.

EXERCISE 1 IN USE OF "I" STATEMENTS

Convert each of the following statements on the left to an "I" statement or to an appropriate "you statement." Suggested answers are given on the right side. Cover them until you have answered.

Nurse's Statement	Transformation
Mr. Jones, you should go back to your room.	Mr. Jones, I want you to go to your room.
It's time for us to get out of bed.	It's time for you to get out of bed.
You are depressed today.	I sense that you are depressed today.
Don't we look nice today.	I think you look really nice today.
(To colleague) You're always late.	It is my perception that you are always late.
You don't make any sense.	I do not understand you.

EXERCISE 2 IN "I" STATEMENTS

1. Pair up.
2. Partners have a conversation about their nursing program or clinical situation using "I" statements and correcting each other if either partner slips up. (You may find yourselves changing sentences like "She's really mean" to "I feel she's really mean.") Pay attention to the differences both as communication sender and receiver to "I" statements.
3. Discuss your reactions in the large group.

Reflection

Reflection is a particularly useful skill in helping a client experience feelings, questions, or ideas. In reflecting, the nurse verbally gives back the feeling parts of the client's communication. Thus, if a client said:

> Client: It's been quite a long day today. They gave me tests and didn't give me results; the doctor hasn't come—it's scary.

An appropriate reflection response is:

Nurse: It's scary for you.

There are two important aspects of this interaction. The first is that the nurse reflects the affective (feeling) words as opposed to answering the implied complaints in the rest of the client's communication. Reflection is a tool to be used to obtain feeling responses, not to exchange information. It will serve to help the client focus and explore his or her own feelings, with the nurse serving as a guide or ally.

By using reflection, the nurse stays with the feeling and ignores extraneous avenues of approach. For example, if the nurse had taken another approach, such as saying, "Why do you feel scared?" (an ineffective technique in itself, as is explained in the following chapter), and the client then proceeded to analyze his or her motives, the result would be quite different from the client continuing to explore the feeling of being scared. Similarly, if the nurse chooses to be reassuring, the feeling level will lighten instead of deepen for the client. Reflection focuses on feelings and tends to result in a deepening of the feeling state as the client responds to the nurse's verbalization and restatement of the client's feelings.

A second major point about reflection is that it can carry with it "unconditional positive regard" for the client (Rogers, 1961). That is, the voice tone, gestures, body posture, and facial expressions of the nurse should be congruent with the message. "You are OK." This empathic response imparts to the client an important covert message of positive self-worth, which can be stronger than a direct verbal message of the same sort. The appropriate message sent by the nurse, then, is not blaming, placating, superreasonable, or irrelevant. It is consistent and focused on the client's self-worth and feeling state at that moment in time.

The following exercises give you an opportunity to practice reflection as a therapeutic tool.

EXERCISE 1 IN REFLECTION

For each of the following statements, think of how you could reflect the feeling words or "tone" of the client's communication. Some possible reflections are included on the right side of the page. (Keep them covered until you think of your answers.)

Client's Statement	Nurse's Reflection
Nurse, what time is it? My sister was supposed to be here an hour ago.	You seem anxious. You're concerned.
I don't feel like doing anything today . . . go away. I'm too upset to talk.	You're too upset to talk?

(Upset) Why are you bothering me? I'm just going to die.	You seem upset. You feel you're going to die?
Why do you want to talk to me?	You sound uncertain.
(Says nothing, just sits and looks out the window—no eye contact.)	You seem distant.
(Sadly) Nobody cares about me. No one knows I'm here.	You seem down.
(Sobbing) I don't know if I'll ever get better.	You feel as if you have no hope?
I'm so worthless.	You feel worthless?

By reflecting feelings in several of these cases, the nurse not only focuses on feelings, but also enables the communication to continue. The focus of the communication is on the client's feelings, not on others—including the nurse. Many times the client will respond directly to the reflection and stop blaming others for his or her feelings. By focusing on the client's feelings, the nurse is keeping the communication in the "here and now," where there is implied hope for change, development of self-worth, or awareness that at least one other person (the nurse) has unconditional positive regard for the client.

EXERCISE 2 IN REFLECTION

Discuss the following questions in the large group:

1. How do you reflect feelings with a relatively uncommunicative client?
2. When is reflection of feeling useful in dealing with other staff, aides, physicians, or other health professionals?
3. When is it awkward *for you* to reflect feelings?
4. Which feelings does it seem hardest to reflect?
5. In which kinds of nursing situations is it easier to use a lot of reflection? In which types is it hardest?
6. How can reflection be misused to keep the nurse from having to answer a difficult question?

Sharing Feelings

Clients in institutional settings are often not allowed to act out feelings in ways that are beneficial to them. Hospitals are relatively inflexible and demand conformity on the part of the client. In addition, the ill client is apt to be immobile. Expressing feelings through verbalization therefore assumes great importance in the institutional setting.

Nurses, to allow for the expression of feelings on the part of clients, must be able to share their own feelings. Along with this goes the ability to observe clients, to decode their behaviors, and to share feelings congruent with the observed behavior while at the same time insuring that the feelings are consistent with the nurse's own behavior. This progression can be summarized with the following hypothetical sequence.

- *Action:* The client is worried about impending operation.
- *Observed behavior of client:* Client clenches jaw, looks anxious, says nothing.
- *Nurse's perception of client's feelings:* Client is fearful about operation.
- *Nurse's communication of own perception and feelings:* "You seem anxious, Mrs. Smith. I feel you are really worried about the operation."
- *Nurse's behavior:* Nurse stands by bed, places hand on client's shoulder.

Nurses who cannot cope with their own feelings about the client may end up "labeling"; that is, instead of eliciting the client's feelings and understanding the client's frame of reference, nurses may make inaccurate assumptions about the client. Consider the following situation:

Mrs. Gifford, a nursing home resident, was found to be hoarding soap. When the nurse looked in her bedside stand, she found 20 bars of soap. The nurse reported to the head nurse: "Mrs. Gifford is selfish!"

The nurse could have elicited Mrs. Gifford's feelings and an explanation of her behavior through a sharing of feelings in this situation. In this instance, it is also important to know that some institutional residents may hoard food or soap as an attempt to be independent, or even to have something to call "one's own."

One important consideration in handling client's feelings is that nurses first understand their own feelings. Nurses cannot help clients to express their feelings without knowing how they themselves react to their own feelings. Do their feelings match their behavior? Are they congruent?

EXERCISE IN SHARING FEELINGS

1. Think how you *act* in the following situations:
   a. When I feel happy I usually _____
   b. When I feel depressed I usually _____
   c. When I feel overworked I usually _____
   d. When I feel fearful I usually _____

    e. When I feel anxious I usually _____
    f. When I feel confident I usually _____
2. Write your responses on paper.
3. Think how you react in each situation. Does your feeling match your action in every situation? Can you detect any incongruent responses in yourself?
4. Now write how clients act in the following situations:
    a. When clients feel anxious they might _____
    b. When clients feel depressed they might _____
    c. When clients feel pain they might _____
    d. When clients feel ignored they might _____
5. Discuss with a partner or share your results with the whole group.

Verbal Reassurance

Along with reflection, a commonly used communication skill is to give verbal reassurance to clients that they are being listened to, that we understand what they say, that good care is being given. By giving reassurance, we play a very important role as a care giver, that of validating the client's self-worth and creating a sense of hope. What one also has to do is to be sure that the reassurance is genuine and truthful. Otherwise we are giving "false reassurance."

What kinds of things, then, can be reassured? A list would include:

- That there is hope
- That one is listening
- That care is available
- That certain disconcerting changes are expected (such as slow recovery from a stroke)
- That the client is being treated like a person
- That the problem is understood

The basic ways in which verbal reassurance can be given include acknowledging any and all of the six points above.

EXERCISE 1 IN VERBAL REASSURANCE

For each of the following situations, think of what you could say to justifiably reassure the client. Some suggested responses are given on the right side of the page. Cover them until you have thought of your own.

Client's Statement	Nurse's Response
My stroke was 4 months ago, and I don't think I'll ever get better.	I know you are concerned, but 4 months is not a long period of

Client's Statement	Nurse's Response
	time for recovery from a stroke.
I don't think anyone here cares what happens to me.	I am here, I care.
I read in the paper that the clinic doesn't have enough money to operate. Can they take care of me?	In any procedures we do in the clinic we use good equipment. While there are some questions about funds, the only way we will stay open is if we can give high quality care.
What difference does it all make? You're just a number here anyway.	I consider you to be a person, Mrs. _____ (be sure you know her name!).

EXERCISE 2 IN VERBAL REASSURANCE

1. Pair up. One partner will be *A*, the other *B*.
2. *B* thinks of a situation in which she as a client might need reassurance.
3. *B* then tells *A* about the situation.
4. *A* and *B* "play out" the communication three times, with *A* as nurse and *B* as client. *A* will reassure *B* each time. *A* will also try different verbal approaches to reassuring *B*.
5. Switch and repeat steps 2–4.
6. Discuss the methods you developed with the rest of the class.

NONVERBAL SKILLS RELATING TO TRUST AND EMPATHY

Four nonverbal skills which nurses can learn to use in order to increase the likelihood of developing an atmosphere of trust and empathy are nonverbal reassurance, attending to the client, active listening, and the use of silence.

Nonverbal Reassurance

Along with verbally expressing reassurance, there are several nonverbal ways the nurse can use to show that the client is cared for and listened to. Nonverbal reassurance refers to everything excluding words that the nurse can do to reassure the client. The use of nonverbal reassurance becomes very important as a subliminal message during the communication sequence, and it should be practiced until it is an active and easily accessible part of the nurse's communication skills.

There are visual, auditory, and kinesthetic ways in which the nurse can reassure the client. Visual ways include the following:

Visual

- Smiling (at the right time)
- Leaning forward
- Nodding head in an affirmative fashion
- Looking concerned (eyebrows down, mouth closed)
- Certain gestures (arms open)
- Maintaining eye contact
- "Open" body stance (arms, legs not crossed)

All of the behaviors in the list indicate "I am receptive to what you have to say" and should serve to reassure clients. It is expected that we will not necessarily do all of these at once, but will practice and learn how to include these symbolic actions as part of our communication repertoire.

Auditory forms of nonverbal reassurance include the following:

Auditory

- Use of "um-humm"
- "Soft" tone of voice
- Relaxed speed of speech
- Allowing the other to finish speaking

The major kinesthetic form of reassurance is, obviously, touch. As mentioned in Chapter 2, there are many ways to touch another. A gentle, reassuring touch can be used to convey nonverbal reassurance in the following ways:

Kinesthetic

- Shaking hands to say hello
- Touching the lower or upper arm
- Touching the shoulder
- Holding the client's hand while communicating
- Hugging from the side (arm around shoulder)
- Frontal hug (pick the *appropriate* time and place)

At this point, a word of caution is offered. Some clients dislike being touched. Nurses must approach touching as a form of nonverbal reassurance carefully. If nurses are not comfortable touching others, and, at the same time, try to convey care primarily through touch, they will transmit incongruent messages. Furthermore, because of the possible sexual overtones to touching in our culture, you may get some surprising responses to touch from clients of the opposite sex. This does not, however, mean you should never give reassurance through touch. Rather, it means you should practice it so that you can communicate quite clearly whatever message *you* want to send.

The following exercises should help you develop and refine your non-verbal reassurance skills.

EXERCISE IN NONVERBAL REASSURANCE

1. Pair up. One partner (*A*) will pretend to be a client with one of the following problems—health problems like diabetes, acne, psoriasis. *A* will describe how the problem affects *A*. The other partner (*B*) will listen to the problem and *visually* show nonverbal reassurance. (*B* can also give verbal reassurance.)
2. Switch roles.
3. *A* will again be the client. This time *B* will add auditory and kinesthetic components of nonverbal reassurance. Experiment with varying degrees of each until you find a good mix that seems to fit you, your partner, and the context of the problem.
4. Switch roles.

Attending to the Client

Effective attending to the client means that the nurses should make sure both the physical arrangement of the space and the nurse's own attention maximize good communication with the client. One would not, for example, want to communicate for a long period of time about personal matters to a client in a wheelchair in the middle of a busy hall while standing up. At the same time, a brief and fairly nonemotion-laden message (e.g., "it's time for lunch") could be adequately communicated in the hall.

There are a few simple points to remember in attending to the client:

- Find a place that is private. This may mean asking a roommate who is not bedridden to leave the room.
- Make sure the client is physically comfortable (in the chair, on the bed, etc.).
- Maximize your ability to hear the client and the client's ability to hear you. Generally, sitting 3 feet apart is recommended.
- Reduce external distractions (close doors, turn off TVs—though be sure to ask first).
- Avoid extensive use of records, charts, questions written on paper, or any other prop that will distract you from the client. Some helpers spend too much time on their notes and no time attending to the client (Brammer, 1988). The client then may feel not listened to.

The second aspect of attending to the client is focusing one's attention to the communication at hand. This is referred to as *physical* attending behavior and implies to the listener that one is there. Postural behaviors such as a forward lean, facing toward the client, and eye contact are attending behaviors. These behaviors can be termed as "immediacy" and not only refer to the closeness between individuals but can be regarded as an index of liking, attention, and openness to the interaction. One study demonstrated that people with high rapport were more likely to be close, to face and lean toward the patient, and to arrange their arms and legs in open postures (Blanck et al., 1986). These nonverbal behaviors show that persons approach what they like and avoid what they dislike through the use of body language.

Nurses seem to show less attending behavior to clients who have terminal illnesses, cancer or are elderly, as well as when they are the bearers of bad news (Mehrabian, 1981). While few nurses would consciously want to convey a "noncaring" attitude to these clients, the relative lack of physical attending behavior may contribute to the sense of despair, depression, and abandonment felt by these client groups.

Active Listening

One of the most effective means of assessing the status of clients is to *listen* to what they tell us. While information on physical and psychological status can be obtained through the different communication channels, what clients state about themselves is most important. Listening then becomes a primary source of communication for nurses.

The levels of hearing and listening were discussed in Chapter 2. Nurses hear multiple messages in the course of their work. This does not mean they have listened to those messages. The average person, after listening to another person talk, remembers only one half of what is heard no matter how much the person was concentrating. In order to listen, nurses must be "actively" engaged in the receiving and decoding or retranslating of the client's message.

Active listening therefore implies that the nurse attends to the content of the message, *how* the client stated the message, and what feelings the client had when the message was stated (Mulhary, 1983). The primary goal of active listening is to understand the situation as the other person sees it—to decode the message in order to recreate the clients' experience within one's own frame of reference.

Nurses who actively listen are able to paraphrase what the client has stated to his or her satisfaction. They are also able to tune into the client's message through observation of body language, eye contact, and nonverbal behavior. In other words, they incorporate all sensory information, including visual, auditory, kinesthetic, and olfactory cues. In addition to receiving communication from all channels, the nurse is actively integrating the information to form a complete picture of the client's emotional state, and this facilitates therapeutic communication. Thus, the nurse is working at all three levels of integration (Level I, sensory; Level II, single channel integration; and Level III, full channel perception).

Active listening is a cognitive process that is developed over a period of time. It is hard work. One of the most effective ways to develop active listening skills is to begin to listen to ourselves. How do we transmit messages? How do we decode a client's message and then verbalize or feed back the decoded message? How effective is our ability to put into our own words what the client has said, as well as letting this client know he or she has been heard? Asking ourselves these questions will enable us to begin to develop the high-level technique of active listening.

Use of Silence

The use of silence is one of the most effective and difficult skills for professional helpers. Often, the nurse has a series of questions to ask. In addition, many interviewers are uncomfortable with even as little as 5 seconds of silence. Somehow they feel nothing is being accomplished if either they or the client is not communicating something at every moment.

Yet silence has many therapeutic uses. It allows the client to dialogue internally and to process information. It also allows time to search for words to describe feelings or situations. Whereas the act of finding "the right words" in and of itself can be therapeutic, allowing the client time to find the words is obviously a useful therapeutic skill.

In most two-way communication, a pattern of responding emerges in which one person talks for a set time, then the other, then the first person, and so on. In terms of therapeutic communication, a silent response coupled with a nonverbal gesture of reassurance, such as a head nod may *allow* the client to continue the train of thought. All that is required is the ability to keep quiet for 5 to 10 seconds. The client will usually pick up his turn.

Obviously, silence can be overused; it can become an excuse for having nothing to say or be the result of tuning out the client. When used judiciously, however, silence is a useful and powerful tool in therapeutic communication. Practice the following exercises until you feel comfortable with silence.

EXERCISE 1 IN USE OF SILENCE

1. Pair up.
2. Sit without talking until you *think* a minute has passed. Check to see how long it has actually been.

EXERCISE 2 IN USE OF SILENCE

1. Pair up.
2. Partner *A* will talk to *B* about an *imaginary* circumstance that makes *A* upset (health, school, family, etc.).
3. *B* will respond, be empathic (as usual), and consciously use silence at three points in the conversation. Take 2–5 minutes.

4. Switch roles.
5. Discuss how it felt to use silence and what thoughts you had as *both* client and interviewer during the silence. What kinds of thoughts emerged? How helpful was the silence?

The communication skills that have been presented are not necessarily effective in all nurse–client interactions. Differences in the use of these skills are reflected through subtle gestures, tone of voice, or expressions. In addition, clients respond in different ways to the same communication skills for a variety of reasons, including channel awareness, "where they are at," and the context in which communication takes place. Effective use of these skills helps to establish an initial rapport between the nurse and the client. Because each client and each nurse are unique, however, it is impossible to give a single specified formula that will indicate what skills should be used in order to create rapport. Some clients may not like attending behavior or reflection statements, while others may prefer nonverbal reassurance and silence. Rapport building can start with a series of "tests" of various skills by nurses to find out which skills work most effectively with a client. Nurses can then become better "guessers" of what will work with a given type of client based on appearance, what clients say, and reports from the nursing staff.

EXERCISE IN ESTABLISHING BEGINNING RAPPORT

1. Form into groups of three. One member will be *A*, one *B*, and one *C*.
2. *A* will role play a client with an emotional reaction to a health problem (e.g., diabetes or hypertension). *B* will be a nurse making a home visit. *B*'s goal is to establish beginning rapport with *A* through the utilization of the four verbal and four nonverbal therapeutic skills presented.
3. Play the scene for 3 minutes. *C* will be an observer and note which skill *B* utilizes, as well as which channel language (visual, auditory, or kinesthetic).
4. At the end of 3 minutes, *C* will review his or her observations. How did the use of skills help (or not help) the development of beginning rapport?

CONCLUSION

Nurses, in order to effectively promote helping relationships, need to develop verbal skills, such as the use of "I" statements, reflection, sharing feelings, and verbal reassurance. Knowledge in the use of nonverbal skills, such as nonverbal reassurance, attending to the client, active listening, and the use of silence, facilitates the nurse's therapeutic use of self and helps to create a sense of trust and empathy in the relationship.

Therapeutic communication is a concept that can be utilized in almost any nursing interaction. Although usually considered crucial in terms of client communication, the opportunity for therapeutic communication with peers or other coworkers may arise. Being therapeutic does not mean the nurse is becoming a junior psychiatrist or psychotherapist. The nurse who is able to respond to others' feelings in a caring manner along with performing other nursing duties is essentially performing at the highest level of the profession.

Yet, therapeutic communication is not the only skill needed by nurses. Nurses need to be able to obtain information, get facts, take histories, and communicate at a content level with clients. The skills nurses use to go about gaining information from clients are the topic of the next chapter on information gathering.

REFERENCES

Alpert, J. S., & Wittenberg, S. M. *A clinician's companion.* Boston: Little, Brown, & Co., 1986.

Barrett-Lennard, G. T. Dimensions of therapist response as causal factors in therapeutic change. *Psychological Monographs,* 1962, 76(43), 562.

Blanck, P. D., Buck, R., & Rosenthal, R. *Nonverbal communication in the clinical context.* University Park, Penn.: Pennsylvania State University Press, 1986.

Brammer, L. *The helping relationship: Process and skills.* (4th ed.). Englewood Cliffs, N.J.: Prentice Hall, 1988.

Brill, E., & Kilts, D. *Foundations for nursing* (2nd ed.). New York: Appleton Century-Crofts, 1986.

Carkhuff, R. *Helping and human relations: A primer for lay and professional helpers* (Vols. I, II). New York: Holt, Rinehart & Winston, 1969.

DiMatteo, R., & Friedman, H. S. *Social psychology and medicine.* Cambridge, Mass.: Oelgeschlager, Gunn, & Hain, 1982.

Gazda, G., Childers, W., & Walters, R. *Interpersonal communication: A handbook for health professionals.* Rockville, Md.: Aspen Systems Corp., 1982.

Janzen, S. A. *Empathic nurse's nonverbal communication.* Doctoral Dissertation (unpublished), University of Illinois, 1984.

Mulhary, T. W. *Interpersonal relations for health professionals: A social skills approach.* New York: MacMillan Publishing Co., 1983.

Rogers, C. R. *On becoming a person.* Boston: Houghton Mifflin, 1961, pp. 39–40.

Schwartz, S., Kogler Hill, S., & Perloff, R. *Interpersonal empathy.* ERIC document 229824, April, 1983.

Sundeen, S. J., Stuart, G. W., Rankin, E. A. & Cohen, S. A. *Nurse–Client interaction* (4th ed.). St. Louis: C. V. Mosby Co., 1989.

Truax, C. B. The process of group therapy: Relationships between hypothesized and therapeutic conditions and intrapersonal exploration. *Psychological Monographs,* 1961, 75 (7), 1–35.

Truax, C. B. Empirical emphasis in psychotherapy: A symposium: Effective ingredients in psychotherapy: An approach to unraveling the patient–therapist interaction. *Counseling Psychology,* 1963, 10, 256–263.

5 Information Gathering Techniques

BEHAVIORAL OBJECTIVES

By reading this chapter and participating in the exercises, students will be able to:

1. Define specific effective information-gathering skills (open-ended questions, appropriate use of focused questions, use of probes, exploring "personal" habits, testing discrepancies, clarification, paraphrasing, summarizing, closing)
2. Apply these skills in an interview
3. Identify common pitfalls in interviews (advice giving, blaming the client, inappropriately changing the topic, defensiveness, false reassurance, judging the client, leading statements, moralizing, multiple questions, overuse of closed-ended questions, parroting, patronizing, placating, rationalizing, stumped silence, "why" questions)
4. Differentiate between effective and ineffective interviewing skills
5. Demonstrate how to transform pitfalls into effective interviewing skills

THE INTERVIEW: AN ASSESSMENT TOOL

This chapter presents some information-gathering techniques related to interviewing in order to enable nurses to process a large volume of information more accurately. A few examples of data to be elicited from clients during the course of an interview are all past and present experiences with illness, how the client interprets the presenting illness, occupational and social roles, level of growth and development, and cultural patterns of daily living.

The nursing history form varies depending on the specific hospital or setting (client's home, hospital, community mental health center, or outpatient clinic, for example). Each history form is designed to elicit essentially the same information, some using open-ended questions and some utilizing checklists. Ideally, when using a checklist type of history form, the nurse should be able to ask questions in such a manner that the client is unaware of the structured nature of the interview. Often nurses develop a format of their own that will allow greater flexibility and adaptability for clients with a variety of problems (Yura & Walsh, 1987).

The purpose of the nursing history, to obtain information, may change during the interview. If the client expresses a need to talk or ventilate feelings, the nurse may want to shift the focus of the interview and utilize those techniques which encourage expression of feelings (see Chapter 4).

The techniques used to obtain information include:

- Asking open-ended questions
- Focusing
- Probing
- Paraphrasing
- Clarifying
- Testing discrepancies (confronting)
- Exploring personal health-related habits (smoking, drinking, medication, or drug use)
- Summarizing
- Closing

Asking Open-Ended Questions

An open-ended question is one that gives the client a wide range of options as to how (and to what) to respond (Enelow & Swisher, 1986). On the other hand, a closed-ended question needs only a one word answer. Open-ended questions are quite useful at the beginning of an interview or at a point where a new topic is being introduced. They allow clients to describe an issue, a feeling, or a problem in their own words, giving as much or as little information as they wish.

Open-ended questions allow clients to describe their personal experience in their own words. Such questions may lead to unexpected yet pertinent information. Many nurses tend to focus too quickly on one problem or an aspect of the problem and miss other equally valuable information that the client has but does not share. An open-ended approach ameliorates the problem of focusing too quickly on one aspect of the client's functioning.

Examples of questions (or implied questions) that are open-ended include:

- How are you today?
- How have you been?
- What brings you in today?
- How is everything going?
- Tell me about (your problem, your family, etc.).
- What seems to be the problem?

A client would have considerable leeway in how to respond to each of these questions.

EXERCISE 1 IN OPEN-ENDED QUESTIONS

Judge each of the following questions. Is it open-ended or closed-ended? When would it be appropriate to ask?

Is 4 o'clock a good time for us to meet?	(Closed)
Do you come here often?	(Closed)
Is the pain in the arm or shoulder?	(Closed)
Is your daughter well?	(Closed)
Doctor, do you think we should ambulate Mr. Jones?	(Closed)
Do you take aspirin for it?	(Closed)
Tell me about your health history.	(Open)
What are you doing for the headache?	(Open)
How have you been?	(Open)
How has your daughter been?	(Open)
Doctor, what should we do for Mr. Jones?	(Open)
When can we meet?	(Open)

EXERCISE 2 IN OPEN-ENDED QUESTIONS

For each of the statements on the left side of the page, think of a more open-ended way to phrase the request. Some suggested alternatives are given on the right side of the page. Cover them until you have answered.

Nurse's Question	Open-Ended Alternative
Where is the pain, when does it hurt, how bad is it?	Tell me about the pain.
Have you been ill this week?	How have you been this week?
Do you have family, brothers, sisters?	Tell me about your family.
You look blue—are you depressed?	You look blue—how are you feeling?
Did you have a good week?	How was your week?

Focusing

A focused question is neither open-ended nor closed-ended but possesses characteristics of both. A focused question limits the area to which the client can respond but still encourages more than a yes or no type of answer. Open-ended questions presented earlier can be considered focused questions if used to pursue a point not covered in the preceding communication. Usually, requests for more information or history about a specific problem can be considered focused questions.

Examples of focused questions include:

- You only mentioned your family briefly. Could you tell me more about them?
- Tell me about the pain in your arm.
- How has the foot been this week?
- You complained of anxiety the last time I saw you. How has it been since then?

EXERCISE IN OPEN-ENDED AND FOCUSED QUESTIONS

1. Form into groups of three. One person will be A, one B, and one C.
2. A will be a client at home. B will be a community health nurse. C will observe.
3. During the conversation C will write down every question B asks.
4. B will begin the dialogue with open-ended questions followed by a few focused questions.
5. At the end of a minute or two, C will tell B how B did.
6. Switch roles until each person has had a chance to take on the three roles.
7. Discuss how focused questions helped the nurse address the issues at hand.

Probing

A probe is any question or statement used to pursue further detail about an area. Thus, focused questions also constitute a beginning probe. Any other phrase, question, or remark the nurse makes to gain further information on the same topic is a probe. Probes can be open-ended, focused, or closed-ended. Some standard probes include:

- Tell me more.
- Can you tell me more?
- Is there anything you left out?
- How do you feel about that?
- And . . .
- Um-hmm (followed by silence).

Probes have to be handled carefully, so they do not seem to be an invasion of the client's sense of privacy. It takes a great deal of practice and sensitivity to be able to determine how far and how much to probe. If you see the client tensing up or hear defensiveness in the client's voice, it may be time to reflect or leave the probe until the client is more relaxed.

EXERCISE IN PROBES

1. Pair up. One partner will be *A*, the other *B*.
2. *A* will give *B* a few sentences about an imaginary health or psychosocial problem.
3. *B* then responds with a probe.
4. *A* then answers the probe. After the answer, *A* will tell *B* how the probe felt, how it could have been improved, and so forth.
5. Switch roles. This exercise is worth doing several times.
6. Discuss the reasons for and against pursuing (probing) issues that are discomforting for the client.

Paraphrasing

Another important skill in interviewing is the ability to paraphrase. Paraphrasing is giving back the client's meaning of a phrase or sentence in your own words. Paraphrasing is similar to reflection in that it is focused on the client's inner process. The major difference is that while reflection attends to feelings, paraphrasing attempts to capture the meaning of what is communicated, be it cognitive or affective.

By using your own words, you are accomplishing two important tasks. First, you are translating the client's words into your own thoughts. Second, you are checking out the translation with the client. This gives the client the opportunity to verify your "translation" and to think further about the matter at hand.

One question that continually arises about paraphrasing is, "How much do I change the words around?" Unfortunately, there is no hard and fast answer. A partial guideline lies in the answer to the following question: "How can I rephrase this so it is in *my* own words?" The answer to this question will vary depending on the nurse, the client, and the context, which are, after all, the three parts of any communication (Satir, 1988).

An example of paraphrasing occurs in the following interaction:

> *Client:* I've had the arthritis for a long time but it doesn't seem to get any worse.
>
> *Nurse:* So, although you've had it quite a while, it's about the same?

Notice that the nurse rephrases "doesn't seem to get any worse" to "it's about the same," which is a reasonable choice. If the rephrasing had been "it's probably better" or "it's hard to tell if it changes," it would not have been a good paraphrase, *even if the client agreed,* because the nurse expanded the client's meaning. Paraphrasing thus becomes a tool to be used carefully in order not to distort the client's meaning.

As is the case for other skills covered in this chapter, one becomes a good "paraphraser" by practicing paraphrasing. The following two exercises are good starting points.

EXERCISE 1 IN PARAPHRASING

For each of the following statements on the left side of the page, think of how you would paraphrase it. That is, how would you say it in your own words without changing the meaning? On the right side of the page are two possible ways of paraphrasing the statement—one acceptable, the other not. Cover them until you have thought of your own.

Client's Statement	Nurse's Paraphrase
I'm originally from California, but I've lived in Florida most of my life.	*Acceptable:* You're originally from the West and have lived in the South. *Not acceptable:* You've moved around a great deal; is that unsettling?
The doctor told me to take one pill three times a day until the pills ran out, but I felt better the next day and stopped.	*Acceptable:* Although the doctor told you to take all the medication, you stopped when you felt better. *Not Acceptable:* You did not understand the doctor.
My child has a 100-degree temperature and has been coughing. What should I do?	*Acceptable:* You need some help on what to do about your child's fever and coughing. *Not acceptable:* That sounds like flu. Don't worry about it.
I haven't been sleeping well. I get up every morning at 3 A.M. and stay awake looking at the ceiling.	*Acceptable:* You've been having trouble sleeping, especially in the morning. *Not acceptable:* Sounds like you're depressed.
I don't believe all this garbage about smoking. I've smoked a pack a day for 35 years with no problems.	*Acceptable:* You're not convinced about the dangers of smoking because they haven't affected you. *Not acceptable:* You won't believe that smoking is

	dangerous until you have a heart attack!
I'd like to lose weight, but you know, the holidays are coming up.	*Acceptable:* You think this is a tough time of year for you to lose the weight you want to.
	Not acceptable: You don't have the will power, that's all.
Nobody in this place gives a damn about you unless you're a private patient.	*Acceptable:* Sounds like you feel you're not being treated like a person here.
	Not acceptable: So you think that getting state aid is accepting charity?

Notice that many of the possible responses by the nurse begin with the word "you." This might seem to be a paradox in light of the discussion in Chapter 4 about the use of "I" statements. A more linguistically correct way to phrase them would be "I think that you. . . ." If this method works for you, use it. Many professionals will use the "you" beginning, assuming that by careful paraphrasing, gestures, facial expression, and voice tone, they will convey the covert message that they are staying with the client's meaning as opposed to judging or interpreting the behavior or words.

EXERCISE 2 IN PARAPHRASING

1. Pair up. One partner will be *A*, the other *B*.
2. Have a discussion about the "highlights of your last week" for 5 minutes using the following rules:
   a. *A* makes a statement (one or two sentences).
   b. *B* has to *paraphrase A*'s statement before responding to it.
   c. *A* has to *paraphrase B*'s response before giving *A*'s next response.
3. Discuss the exercise in a large group using the following questions as guides:
   a. How much "work" is it to paraphrase?
   b. When is paraphrasing *appropriate* in nursing communication?
   c. When is paraphrasing *inappropriate* in nursing communication?
   d. Did anyone get so absorbed in the paraphrasing that they forgot what they were going to say next?

Clarifying
Often, a client will say or do something in the course of an interview that the nurse does not understand. When this occurs, there is an immediate question

of judgment that has to be answered: "Do I need to understand this now?" If the answer is that you do, then a request for clarification is appropriate. Other choices can include requesting clarification later on (especially if the client is quite upset and not listening too well) or in a subsequent interview.

If the request for clarification is presented with warmth and empathy, it is likely to be perceived by the client as a sign of interest and an honest attempt to create understanding. It also "models" asking for clarification, and hopefully the client can use the same skill with the interviewer.

There are many ways to request clarification. Some examples include:

- I'm not sure I understood that completely. Could you repeat it?
- I missed the last few words you said.
- I don't follow you. Can you say it another way?

EXERCISE IN CLARIFICATION

1. Pair up. One partner will be *A*, the other *B*.
2. *B* will be the client, *A* the nurse. *B* will think of a confusing sentence to say to *A*, such as:
   Things are so nice here, I feel so terrible.
   So you're the nurse who doesn't like me.
   The idea is to confuse *A*.
3. *A* will respond by asking for clarification.
4. Repeat this two times and then switch roles. If you are having trouble thinking of confusing statements, think about all the confusing things that have been said to you in the last week. You should have no problem finding one that fits the nurse–client setting.
5. In the large groups, share your experiences from the pairs, including the "most confusing statements" and listing all the ways members of your group seek clarification.

Testing Discrepancies

In many interviews, there will be information, feelings, explanations, and even body language expressed by the client that are not consistent. For example, a male client with tears in his eyes may deny his feelings by saying, "I feel fine." Or, an older client in a nursing home might at one point tell you that the family visits every day and then later complain of feeling lonely. Neither of these instances is congruent; that is, the messages do not make sense when put together. The question then is, "What do I, the nurse, do about this?"

Discrepancies such as the ones given above can be categorized into two groups: "incongruity of message" and "conflict of information." Incongruity of message refers to an inconsistency between the words, tone, gestures, and body language of the client in a single message. Conflict of information means that the data presented by the client at one moment in time differ from that presented at another.

When the nurse notes a discrepancy, a decision has to be made about what to do. There are basically three choices: ignore it, explore it, or note it for further probing at a later time. The following exercise should help you begin to develop strategies for exploring discrepancies in your client's behavior.

EXERCISE IN TESTING DISCREPANCIES

For each of the situations on the left side of the page, think of a way you could verbally explore the discrepancy with the client. Suggested answers are on the right side of the page. Cover them until you have thought of your answers.

Client's Discrepancy	Nurse's Response
A client sits in a health clinic, eyes wandering and generally distracted. When asked how he feels, he says, "Just fine."	You say you're just fine, but your eyes and body seem tense. I'm confused about how you really feel. (Use of "I" statement)
An older person gives you two different numbers on the same street as his address.	You just gave me another number a few minutes ago. Do you know which one is correct?
A mother complains about her child's behavior with a slight grin on her face.	I'm sure you're upset, and I notice smiling at the same time. How does that fit?
A hospitalized client comments on the frequency of family visits. Later the client admits to feeling lonely "all of the time."	You say you're lonely all of the time. Before you told me that the family visits often. How do you make sense out of that?
A client claims to never get drunk, yet complains of blackouts, poor attendance at work, and bad headaches in the morning.	To what do you attribute the blackouts and the problems at work?

These situations are not easy ones. Yet, they are common. After you have finished the exercise, discuss the following related questions in a large group.

- How can you approach an older person about a memory problem with respect and a professional attitude?
- How much can you challenge an alcoholic or a mother who gives conflicting messages to children *without losing the client* (important for community health work)?

- If you explore the discrepancy and the client cannot "explain" it, what can you do? Do you have to do anything?

Exploring Personal Health-Related Habits

One area of interviewing that gives many new nurses difficulty is asking questions about "personal" information. Personal information includes areas which the culture considers private, taboo, or not to be discussed openly. In health settings, "loaded" topics that need to be discussed include alcohol consumption, smoking, drug usage, and sexual functioning.

The aspect of these topics that distinguishes them from other areas that might create anxiety for a client is that the nurse may feel that even broaching the area is an invasion of privacy, given the cultural taboos. The nurse may therefore gloss over these areas, not probe effectively, or fail to reflect feelings, even though the topic may be one in which the client needs the most help. The nurse needs to be as comfortable as possible in discussing these areas, being able to put aside personal feelings so as to be capable of responding empathically to the client while at the same time obtaining the needed information. It is helpful for some nurses to realize that these areas are being discussed in a professional, confidential setting for the benefit of the client. To ignore or obtain inadequate information in these areas could have detrimental effects for the client and thus be a disservice rather than a sign of respect for the client's privacy.

Keeping these thoughts in mind, an initial criterion for approaching these areas during an interview is that a sense of trust and respect should have been developed between the nurse and client using the information given in the previous chapter. It would be most awkward, for example, to start an interview by immediately getting into serious health concerns without any "warm-up" or relationship building, even if the relationship building aspects last only a few moments.

Assuming an atmosphere of trust has been established, how does one raise the issue of drinking, smoking, sex, and drug use? As noted, these can be sensitive areas. The manner in which the issue is raised is as important as the way in which the questions or requests are phrased. Several of the authors referred to in this book (e.g., Rogers, 1951; Satir, 1988) imply that the nurse convey (by manner, posture, voice tone, breathing rate, facial expression, and rate of speech) that anything the client says or does in response to these questions is OK. A sense of unconditional acceptance for the client will yield much more useful information in these areas than a stern, judgmental, anxious, or moralizing manner.

In a sense, once an atmosphere of trust and acceptance has been established, asking questions about sex, smoking, drinking, and drug use is like talking about any other topic. Begin with open-ended or focused questions, followed by probes, requests for clarification, and summation. A healthy dose of verbal and nonverbal reassurance is quite useful, since many clients will be struggling to find the words to describe private and occasionally frightening experiences.

In addition, the following focused/closed-ended questions can be useful as lead-in statements to personal areas of functioning:

- *Drinking:* Do you ever take a drink?
- *Smoking:* Do you smoke?
- *Drugs:* Have you ever used drugs? What medication do you take?
- *Sex (for adolescents):* Do you have a boy/girl friend? How do you spend your time together?
- *Sex (for adults):* How do you and your (partner, wife, husband, etc.) spend your time together? What's the nature of your sexual relationship?

After any of the lead-ins, watching and listening carefully to the client's response allow the nurse to quickly evaluate the direction in which the interview should proceed: more information (probes, focused questions), empathy (reflection, verbal/nonverbal reassurance), or temporarily leaving the topic. In choosing the latter case, a comment by the nurse about the situation (metacomment) is reassuring, such as "I see that this is uncomfortable for you. Should we come back to this later?"

EXERCISE 1 IN INTERVIEWING ABOUT PERSONAL ISSUES

Below is part of a hypothetical dialogue between a nurse and client. Assume they have been talking for 10 minutes at a high school health clinic. The client is a 16-year-old girl. After each statement by the client, think about what you would say or do. Then read the nurse's response and the type of skill/questioning procedure used. Are there any options that are better than the ones suggested?

> *Client:* So that's why I came in. I'm having trouble sleeping and wondered if you could get me anything for it?
>
> *Nurse:* Um-hmm, could you tell me about your social life? (Lead-in)
>
> *Client* (looks down, fidgets, blushes): Well, I haven't gone out too much with guys, if that's what you mean.
>
> *Nurse:* And? (Tone of voice reassures; "and" serves as a *gentle probe*)
>
> *Client:* Well, there's this one guy I met at a basketball game a few months ago from another school.
>
> *Nurse:* Sounds like you liked him. (Reflects)

Client: I did, but we went out a few times without my parents' knowing about it; then they found out and wouldn't let me see him again. They said he's the "wrong type for me."

Nurse: How did you spend your time together? (Focuses, leads in)

Client: We went to a few parties, drank a little.

Nurse: Do you remember how much you drank at the parties? (Probe)

Client: Oh—you mean did I get drunk? (Giggles) Well, once I drank two beers and felt light-headed, but that was it.

Nurse: Have you been drinking since then? (Probe)

Client: No, I really didn't like it.

Nurse: Were there any drugs at the parties? (Said in empathetic, understanding, professional tone. Lead-in)

Client: Are you gonna tell?

Nurse: I'm concerned primarily with you right now (Reassures). What I do with the information depends on what it is.

Client: Well, one night a couple of kids were passing a cigarette around—I'm not sure, but it *could* have been a joint.

Nurse: Did you try it? (Probe)

Client (agitated): Just don't tell my folks any of this. They'd kill me.

Nurse: You seem scared of your parents. (Reflects and changes focus)

Client: It's terrible. Whenever I come home, I get the third-degree. "Where'd you go, what did you do, with whom, be careful"—it's awful.

Nurse: Are you doing anything with your boyfriend that they would be concerned about? (Lead-in)

Client: Like what?

Nurse: Are you sexually involved? (Probe)

Client: Oh, that. No, I mean we kissed and all that, and they would be concerned about that, believe you me.

Nurse: Although I'm not sure about your own use of drugs, I know you've drunk a little, you're not sexually involved with your boyfriend, but you're having some hassles with your parents. (Summarizes) Is that right?

Client: That's it, but I don't use drugs, I don't even smoke. Just please don't tell my folks I've been at a party where there were drugs. They'd *kill* me.

After you have read and thought through the scenario, discuss the following questions:

1. How much probing was appropriate?
2. Could you, as a nurse, do this sort of interview keeping your personal values separate from your professional role?

3. How could you have given reassurance without "taking sides" on the issues?
4. Of all these issues (sex, drugs, alcohol), which are easiest for you to discuss? Can you think of ways to begin to make the difficult areas easier for you to handle with clients?

EXERCISE 2 IN INTERVIEWING ABOUT PERSONAL ISSUES

1. Form into groups of three. One person will be *A*, one *B*, and one *C*.
2. *A* will be a client at a health screening clinic. *B* will be the interviewer. Pretend you have been talking a few minutes, have developed rapport, etc. *B* will then do a lead-in (focused or open-ended question) and probe for each of the following topics; *C* will write down *B*'s questions as *B* asks them.
   a. Smoking
   b. Drinking
   c. Medication
   d. Drugs
   e. Sexual activity
3. At the end of these questions, *C* (who should have observed the communication) will comment on how *B* did, that is how the questions sounded: did *B* seem relaxed, what gestures were used, and what was the body language? *A* will also comment on how it felt to be asked the questions by *B*.
4. Switch roles so each person gets to be the client, the interviewer, and the observer.

Summarizing

At the end of an interview or at a logical breaking point in an interview, many effective nurse communicators find it useful to summarize what the client has said. Summarizing means verbally capturing the essence of what the client presented including pertinent facts, feelings, discrepancies, and untouched areas (Brammer, 1988). Consider the following example:

A nurse has been talking with a 46-year-old male who is getting ready for hospital discharge following a heart attack. The discussion has included a review of his recovery plan, including exercise and diet, as well as his perceptions of the family's response to his illness. He has also voiced concerns about his sexual functioning to the nurse, but not to his wife and has openly wondered about what the effect of all of this will be on his work as a vice-president of an advertising agency.

One way of briefly summarizing all of this is as follows:

"Let me see if I have everything we talked about. We have reviewed your recovery plans and your family's reaction to the heart attack. You still have some concerns about its effects on your work at the advertising agency and on your sexual relationship with your wife, although you have not yet discussed this with her. Is there anything else?"

The purpose of summarization is threefold. First, it forces you, the nurse, to pull pieces of the interview together for future recording. Second, the client has a sense that the nurse has understood what has been said, which is a good rapport building experience. Third, the client has a chance to review the information and add any missing pieces. Many clients wait until the last minute to give nurses the most important information (e.g., "By the way, I've been having slight chest pain," in the type of case presented above). Summarization makes a logical place for this information to emerge.

The following exercise is one way to begin thinking about summarization.

EXERCISE IN SUMMARIZING

For each of the "case notes" on the left side of the page, figure out how you could summarize the "interview" in one or two sentences. A suggested summary is given on the right side of the page. Cover it until you have figured out your own.

Cases	Summary
1. A female client came to a health clinic upset over migraine headaches. She had gone to three doctors over the last 2 years who "do nothing." The client had just been fired from a job she needed to support two children. At the time, she smoked two packs of cigarettes a day.	As I understand it, you have had migraine headaches for a while, but the physicians you have seen have not helped. You also have to support your two children and currently have no job.
2. An elderly man's blood pressure was found to be elevated at a health screening clinic. He said he had medicine but did not take it because he felt	Your blood pressure is high. You've had it before but you don't take the medicine because you feel all right. You haven't recently checked with your physician.

OK. He hadn't been to a doctor in a year.

3. A postoperative phlebitis client feels tired but hopeful of fast recovery. Her husband has not been in to see her, and she expresses worry over where he is.

From what you've said, you're still feeling the effects of the operation. You would like to get on your feet soon and are concerned that your husband has not been in to visit you in the hospital.

Closing

Along with summarizing at the end of the interview, the nurse should give the client a sense that the time has come for the interview to end. This is important when the interview is time-bound; for example, when there are usually other clients waiting, closure should be done smoothly so the client feels finished as opposed to cut off.

One way of doing this includes acknowledging the end of the interview and the time spent with the client, as in "Well, I see our time is nearly up. It's been really nice talking with you today." Other statements that could be made are:

- I have to finish in a minute.
- We need to wrap up now.
- That's about all the time I have—would you like another appointment?

PITFALLS OF INTERVIEWING: COMMON WAYS OF HINDERING COMMUNICATION

Up to this point, the focus of this chapter has been on effective strategies, tools, and techniques with which the nurse can perform a successful interview. "Effective" suggests that the way in which the communication is given is respectful of the client's and nurse's self-worth, that the content message is clear, that the communication promotes trust and that the client has a maximum opportunity to express his or her own feelings or views without being overly influenced by the nurse.

The aspects of effective interviewing mentioned earlier in this chapter meet all of these requirements. The "pitfalls" enumerated below do not.

Pitfalls in communication are strategies, styles, or techniques that are non-therapeutic; they create distrust and restrict the response of the client. Non-therapeutic communication leads to decreased self-worth of either the client or nurse.

We all use nontherapeutic techniques at various times when we communicate with others. An awareness of our use of these pitfalls is the first step toward more effective communication interaction with clients. Sixteen pitfalls are presented in alphabetical order in this section; and although there is overlap between some pitfalls, each will be discussed separately.

Pitfall 1—Giving Advice

Giving advice on advice giving is relatively simple: *don't!* There are several reasons for limiting advice giving in a clinical setting. The first is that the advice generally will not be taken. The second is that if the client "takes it to heart," the nurse who gave the advice may be blamed if anything goes wrong. And the third reason is that clients are likely to misinterpret the advice and not follow it carefully.

What exactly is advice? The dictionary defines it as an opinion. When clients ask nurses for an opinion or advice about what to do, the nurse may well (inadvertently) set him- or herself up to take inappropriate responsibility for clients' decisions. If it is a question of an "informal nursing opinion," nurses can use the tactic of giving clients information and exploring options as opposed to giving advice. The client is viewed as an active participant in the health process; for this reason the giving of advice is not advocated.

The following statements on the left side of the page represent advice. Some non-advice ways of rephrasing the statements are on the right.

Advice	Preferred
If you want my opinion, I think you should . . . (in situation where client has two choices).	What are the pros and cons of each choice for you?
You've just got to try harder, that's all.	What is holding you back?
Anyone can see that the way to discipline is	What are some ways you could try to discipline the child?
Generic drugs are better than brand names.	Do you know the difference between generic and brand name drugs?
My advice is—go on a diet.	How can you lose the weight you need to?

There is also occasionally a context in which it is appropriate for nurses to make suggestions. When this happens, ideally the suggestion should be presented as another option clients can consider along with any others. It can sometimes be difficult for nurses to allow clients maximum responsibility for their own choices because nurses' power as authorities in the clinical context may influence those choices.

Pitfall 2—Blaming the Client

Blaming was presented in Chapter 3 as an ineffective communication style. Blame carries with it decreased self-regard for the client who is directly or indirectly being told "It's your fault." There is, however, a subtle but important distinction between blame and responsibility.

Clients can be responsible for many aspects of their own health and well-being. They can be educated as to how certain aspects of their lives led up to their current state of health (eating, exercise, life style, job pressure, smoking, drinking, etc.). When the educational aspect turns into a put-down and an implied message of accusation, then the client will feel blamed and guilty and experience lowered self-worth. Along with these nontherapeutic aspects of blaming, most psychological research has demonstrated that simple punishment—for example, blaming—is not an effective way to change behavior. What often happens is that only certain patterns of behavior change; the client will stop coming to the clinic or making appointments, for example. In this way the client avoids blame and punishment.

Blame can also come under the guise of advice. There are an infinite number of ways to blame the client. Some are obvious, some not. Many are unintended. Some examples of blame are:

- Well, you should have called earlier to make an appointment.
- Don't you know that smoking is bad?
- You're supposed to eat everything on your plate.
- Look, we told you to take your medication three times a day. What's the matter with you?

One way to work on blaming behavior is first identifying it in ourselves and then transforming it into a message that indicates respect for ourselves as well as clients. The following exercise is a step in that direction.

EXERCISE IN BLAME TRANSFORMATION

For each of the following blame statements on the left side of the page, first say it out loud and add appropriate voice and facial expression to make it blaming. Then change the statement (or the tone and expression) so it still conveys the correct content but also respects the self-worth of the client. Say this "transformation" out loud. If you cannot think of one, use the suggested transformation on the right side of the page.

Blame Statement (remember to say these with appropriately blaming tone)	Transformation
What are you doing out of bed?	You're supposed to be in bed. What's the problem?
Why haven't you been here for your last two appointments?	I see you missed two appoint- What happened?
What have you done to your child?	What happened to the child?
Why haven't you eaten your dinner?	You haven't eaten your dinner.

	(Change of voice tone is important.)
You should have this checked immediately.	This should be checked immediately.

Pitfall 3—Changing Topic Inappropriately

A third common pitfall in nursing communication is the inappropriate change of topic by the nurse. This is related to Satir's concept of "irrelevancy" discussed in Chapter 3. Generally, nurses change topics inappropriately more as a result of their own rising anxiety than for reasons specifically related to clients. Thus, the change of topic is inappropriate in that it is not a strategy that helps clients.

If nurses find themselves inappropriately changing topics while interviewing clients, an investigation of the following areas might help to suggest the source of their anxiety.

- The client is touching on a topic area about which the nurse feels uncomfortable (sex, emotional problems).
- The nurse is unsure of what to do and is uncomfortable just listening.
- The client is describing a problem that exists for the nurse.
- The nurse is embarrassed by what the client says.

Pitfall 4—Defensiveness

Defensiveness is a more general category than many of the other pitfalls reviewed in this chapter. As you may recall from Chapter 3, defensiveness is defined as "being hostile, aggressive, not listening, or responding as if one had been attacked." There are times when any nurse will feel defensive, be it triggered by something that happened at home, on the job, or during the interview. There are two schools of thought on what to do at these times. One is to finish the interview as if "nothing is the matter" and then work things through with a head nurse or supervisor.

The second school of thought is to comment on one emotional state *briefly* to the client. Giving the client some understanding about how you, the nurse, are acting. Examples of how to acknowledge your own defensiveness briefly include:

- I feel somewhat uncomfortable about this topic but I am listening to you carefully.
- I want to let you know I'm upset by other things today. Please do not take my reactions as a statement about you.

There are reasons to share *and* not share one's own defensiveness with clients. The reasons for sharing include the following:

- Models self-disclosure
- Explains own behavior
- Can build trust
- Helps nurse to get over the defensiveness

The reasons for not sharing one's own defensiveness include the following:

- Client could be overwhelmed.
- It could be taken as a sign of weakness or incompetence.
- The nurse could end up "being the client."
- Clients can feel pressured into disclosing things they are not ready to disclose.

Pitfall 5—False Reassurance

One of the great temptations to any nurse is to "lighten the emotional load" of a distressed client. Ways in which an effective nurse communicator can give appropriate verbal and nonverbal reassurance have already been discussed in Chapter 4. There are times when, with good intentions, the nurse gives false reassurance. That is, in trying to reassure the client, the nurse promises something that may not happen, says something that is untrue, or provides comfort in an incongruent manner. Examples of the three forms of false reassurance are:

1. Promising something that may not happen: "Don't worry. Everything will be all right."
2. Saying something not true: "You have nothing to worry about."
3. Giving incongruent comfort: "I feel for you" (when in actuality, the nurse is trying to figure out what to do next).

False reassurance may raise clients' anxiety. Rather than being reassured, the client will become suspicious and more concerned as the inconsistency in the message from the nurse is noted. By inconsistency, we mean that either the nurse's message is incongruent or it is inconsistent with the client's perception of the problem.

EXERCISE IN IDENTIFYING AND TRANSFORMING FALSE REASSURANCE

For each of the following statements, decide if it is either "false" or "true" reassurance. If it is false, figure out a way to make it more congruent.

Answers and suggested transformations are given on the right side of the page.

Nurse's Statement	Type of Reassurance
I hear what you are saying. You seem to feel hopeless.	Reassurance.
Don't worry. Everything will work out for the best.	False reassurance. Transformation: You seem worried. Is there anything I can do?
Look, it's not so bad. I've seen patients in worse shape than this who have gotten better.	False reassurance. Transformation: I think you have every reason to hope for the best.
It's OK to cry when you feel like it.	Reassurance.
There's no need to cry. It's not the end of the world, is it?	False reassurance. Transformation: It's OK to cry. I'll wait for you.
(Edgily) Sure, tell me about it.	False reassurance. Transformation: Other things are bothering me. Let me get collected. OK, what's the problem?

Pitfall 6—Judging the Client

Judging the client incorporates any tendencies the nurse has to evaluate the client as being "good" or "bad." In general practice, more emphasis is put on negative evaluation of the client than positive evaluation, however, even positive evaluation (as opposed to *unconditional* positive regard) can have problems. For example, if nurses are in the habit of nodding their heads and saying "that's good" during an interview when they hear things they like, clients will quickly learn to tell only those things that get rewarded and they may leave out pertinent information concerning their health.

There is an important distinction that needs to be made between evaluating *behavior* and evaluating the *client*. For example, it is quite appropriate to tell a client that a self-administered procedure was done incorrectly. That is your job. There can be, however, negative consequences if the message carries with it a negative judgment of the client as well. Most clients respond to "being judged" by becoming uncooperative.

A client can feel judged by seeing a raised eyebrow, a "stern" look, hearing a raised voice, or by being blamed. In all fairness, clients may feel judged even when no judgment is intended or made. Since the client is likely to be extremely sensitive to judgment, it is important to take note of all the ways nurses can judge the client and work on developing nonjudgmental communication.

EXERCISE IN JUDGING THE CLIENT

This exercise is designed to help you discover ways in which you and other nurses can come across as judgmental, as well as to give you ways to change your own judgmental communication.

1. Pair up. One partner will be *A*, one *B*.
2. *A* will read the following list of paired statements to *B*. Read the first statement in a judgmental tone, using judgmental gestures, facial expressions, etc. Be expressive and creative; then read the paired statement (which will either be reworded or remain the same) in a nonjudgmental manner.

Judgmental	Nonjudgmental
You don't take good care of your child.	Raising a child alone is difficult.
I would never do that.	What prompted you to do that?
You're stupid to eat sweets with your diabetes.	I would like to talk with you about your diet.
I see you're late for your appointment.	I see you're late for your appointment.
If you weren't so depressed people would like you.	Have you ever thought that people may react to how you are feeling?
Your husband has no manners.	How do you feel about your husband?
Hello, I'm your nurse. How are you today?	Hello, I'm your nurse. How are you today?

3. Switch roles and do step 2 again.
4. Discuss how it felt to receive the judgmental and nonjudgmental statements.

Pitfall 7—Leading Statements

A common mistake of beginning interviewers is to "put words in the client's mouth" or make a leading statement. A leading statement is any one that indirectly makes the *interviewer's* interpretation or observation appear to be the client's. Several examples include:

- You're tired because you're depressed, right?
- You probably forgot the appointment because you were worried about the holidays.
- It doesn't hurt too much, does it?

The problem with a leading statement is that it does not give the client a full opportunity to decide if it is true or not, especially if the client is under stress.

EXERCISE IN LEADING STATEMENTS

Identify the effective interviewing strategies and leading statements by the nurse in the following interview. The type of statement is given on the right side of the page. Keep it covered until you have decided.

Client: Well, I just do not know how my husband will adjust to me recovering from this stroke. He spends time with me—but doesn't say much. I don't know what he's thinking.

Nurse: You say you're not sure about your husband's reaction.　Paraphrase
You seem concerned.　Reflection
How long has he been upset?　Leading

Client: Well. I had the stroke 2 months ago. He had to work and I was in no shape to talk, if you catch my drift. My arm still feels stiff. Anyway, he started to spend time with me 1 month ago.

Nurse: I can understand how you and he don't know if you're ever going to get better.　Leading ("Know if you're *ever* going to get better")

What brought about the change in his behavior?　Probe

You will notice that the client does not necessarily respond directly to the leading statements. Also, the second leading statement, which was an attempt to reflect, could serve to plant or exaggerate an unsurfaced fear the client has. The way it is presented makes it difficult for the client to verbalize her own fears.

Pitfall 8—Moralizing

Moralizing is a specific form of judging the client. While there is no exercise on moralizing presented here, it is worthy of comment. Moralizing refers to any instance in which nurses judge clients based on their own personal values. Examples of moralizing statements include:

- How can you smoke at your age?
- Why do you eat sugar when you are overweight?
- Abortion is sinful.
- Abortion is OK for everyone.

A good question for discussion is: "How can I be an effective nurse with someone whose values differ significantly from mine on the issue at hand?"

Pitfall 9—Multiple Questions

A less emotionally charged pitfall is use of multiple questions. Multiple questions are really a series of questions that are asked as if they were one question. For example:

- Did you forget the appointment or did you have something else or did you call and the line was busy?
- Where do you live—is it an apartment and what is your neighborhood like?

Multiple questions are difficult to answer. Clients, especially when distressed, can easily get confused as to which question should be answered first. Many multiple questions get asked because the nurse is somewhat anxious and does not give the client adequate time to think of a response. The nurse assumes that the client is having a problem figuring out the question, and, without checking it out, asks another question (or two). The result can be confusing.

Any multiple question can be broken down into separate single questions that can then be posed to the client. In other words, nurses can ask one question at a time and wait for the client to respond before rephrasing or asking another question.

EXERCISE IN MULTIPLE-QUESTION TRANSFORMATION

Transform each of the multiple questions on the left side of the page into a separate question. Make the initial one open-ended. A suggested breakdown is given on the right side of the page. Keep it covered until you have decided how to separate the questions.

Multiple Question	Transformation
Did you sleep well, enjoy breakfast, and have a good morning?	How was last night? (Wait) How was breakfast? (Wait) How has the morning been? (Wait)

Multiple Question	Transformation
Tell me about your family, your work, your hobbies so I can get to know you.	Tell me about your family. (Wait) Can you tell me about your work? (Wait) What kind of hobbies do you have? (Wait)
What caused the problem? Was it stress, diet, exercise or something you ate? (This is also a leading question.)	How did the problem come about? (Note: Only one question is necessary here.)

Pitfall 10—Overuse of Closed-Ended Questions

As mentioned earlier, closed-ended questions elicit one or two word responses. Obviously, there are certain closed-ended questions that are appropriate, such as requests for specific information (name, address, names of medication, etc.). However, these direct questions can be overused when the purpose of the communication is to open up a new area or probe further into a relatively unexplored one.

For example, a nurse who wants to explore an older person's drug use and "chooses" to use direct-closed-ended questions will come out with a series of questions such as the following:

Nurse	Client
Do you take any medication?	Yes.
Are any prescribed?	Yes.
Do you have some for your heart?	Yes.
For your blood pressure?	Yes.
Do you take a laxative?	Sometimes.
Does it work?	Sometimes.
What is it?	Why are you asking me all these questions?

By overusing closed-ended questions, the nurse becomes an interrogator, puts the client on the defensive, and has to do most of the talking. Except in the case where there is a checklist of items to be asked, open-ended questions, such as, "Tell me about your medication," followed by *appropriate* focused and occasional closed-end probes can be a more effective approach.

EXERCISE IN CLOSED-ENDED QUESTIONS

Change each series of closed-ended questions on the left side of the page to a more general open-ended question. A suggested answer is on the right side of the page. Keep it covered until you have thought of your answer.

Closed Questions	Open Question
SERIES 1	
Do you live in a house?	Tell me about your living
By yourself?	arrangements.
Do you have pets?	
What kind?	
How many rooms?	
SERIES 2	
Where is the pain?	Tell me as much about the pain
How much does it hurt?	as you can.
Does it hurt at night?	
By day?	
How did it start?	
SERIES 3	
Do you have brothers, sisters?	I'd like to know about your family.
Are you married, how long?	
Is your relationship with your	
spouse good?	
Do you have children?	
SERIES 4	
Do you eat a good breakfast?	What kinds of food do you eat in
How much coffee or tea do you	a normal day?
drink?	
Do you eat dessert? Which ones?	
Do you eat a balanced diet?	

Pitfall 11—Parroting

"Parroting" refers to the continual repetition of parts of the client's phrases as an attempt to reflect or paraphrase. While occasional repetition of portions of the phrases is effective in highlighting aspects the nurse would like the client to pursue, the overuse of this technique makes the nurse seem like a parrot, mechanically repeating whatever is said.

The following dialogue shows how parroting is used. Reflective statements are included in parentheses:

Client	Nurse
I'm concerned about my son.	You're concerned about your son. (Reflect: You seem upset.)
He seems to be losing weight.	He's losing weight. (Reflect: You're concerned about his weight.)

Client	Nurse
He stays out all night.	He stays out. (Reflect: You're concerned.)
He has tremors and I don't know what to do about him.	You don't know what to do. (Reflect: You feel unsure about what to do.)

Pitfall 12—Patronizing the Client

Often, nurses and other health professionals talk to elderly clients and children in an overly kind manner, as if the client needed to be "talked down to" or put on a lower level than the helper or nurse. It is not so much a matter of words but how the words are said that gives the impression that clients are being treated as if they were less than human. The words and voice tones are not hostile; they are, if anything, too sweet.

Patronizing the client refers to any and all ways the client is talked down to while being comforted. Several communication patterns that go along with patronizing the client include the nurse's keeping his or her eye level higher than that of the client (for example, standing while the client is sitting), talking in a sing-song voice, using "we" when either "you" or "I" is meant, and using (for lack of a better term) "baby talk" words, phrases, or voice tone.

The results of patronization are lowered self-worth and increased dependence (or anger) by the client. There is no valid reason to patronize a client. Even though the nurse may be patronizing unintentionally, all clients deserve to be treated as equals in the interaction.

EXERCISE IN PATRONIZATION

This exercise is designed to help you learn how you could come across when you are patronizing.

1. Pair up. One partner will be A, the other B.
2. A will say each of the three statements below and be as patronizing as possible. After each statement B will then repeat it exactly as A did, with similar voice tone, gestures and facial expressions. A will closely attend to B to find out how A came across.
   a. How are you today?
   b. It's time for us to get out of bed.
   c. Oh, you didn't eat your lunch. Is something the matter?
3. Switch roles and repeat.
4. Discuss the following questions in the large group.
   a. Have you ever seen anyone be patronizing in a nursing context?
   b. What was the effect of it?
   c. What would have been needed to help that person change? Who should have been involved (superior, client, peers, etc.)?

Pitfall 13—Placating the Client

A pitfall that is related to being patronizing is placating. Placating is one of Satir's communication categories referred to in Chapter 3. Placating the client means that the nurse agrees with everything, takes the blame for everything, and cannot say no. Placating does not mean unconditional regard for the client.

The results of placating the client include decreased self-worth for the nurse, as well as either dependence or anger on the part of the client. The temptation to placate can exist, however, when it is easier to say yes to a demanding client than to say no and have to defend oneself.

For an exercise on placating, refer to the other exercises in Chapter 3.

Pitfall 14—Rationalizing Feelings

Rationalizing feelings means finding an apparently reasonable excuse for having the feelings. In fact, the excuse is not reasonable; it is an attempt to explain away whatever is being felt. This form of pitfall is a result of being "superreasonable" at a moment in time. Superreasonable is another of Satir's defensive communication styles. It refers to using reasons to protect the self from uncomfortable feelings.

When rationalization is used, then, the nurse is probably feeling anxious. Some examples of rationalizing phrases are:

- Oh, well, that's probably because . . .
- It's not important because . . .
- Everyone feels a little . . .
- I misunderstood you because I thought you were done.

The problem with rationalization is that feelings and behavior are subtly dismissed (e.g., "I only did that because . . ."). Rationalization also eliminates some of the unpleasant truths about the motivation for behavior in an interview, however, to rationalize the avoidance of a sensitive topic clouds the reason for discontinuing, since it may be the nurse's problem, not the client's.

The following exercise is designed to help nurses begin to recognize rationalization and transform it to a more accurate statement of reality.

EXERCISE IN RATIONALIZATION TRANSFORMATION

In each of the following communications, identify the nurse's rationalization. Then, change the nurse's rationalization to a more accurate statement of feelings or observation of what is going on with the client. Suggested answers are given on the right side of the page. Cover them until you have made your own.

STATEMENT 1

Client: I've never talked about this problem. I'm not sure you can help me. It's private.

Nurse: I see. I'd like to help. You probably never talked about it because you were afraid. You do not have to worry.

Rationalization: Because you were afraid.

Transformation: It's been hard for you to talk about it. (Reflection)

STATEMENT 2

Client: I've gained 25 pounds with this pregnancy. I read somewhere that you should only gain 15 to 20 pounds at my weight. What should I do?

Nurse: I wouldn't worry. It was probably an uninformed opinion. What have you been eating?

Rationalization: I wouldn't worry (because it was probably an uninformed opinion).

Transformation: You seem concerned. Would you like me to find out more on this for you?

STATEMENT 3

Client: So I took grandfather home from the hospital and then, one night, he began to . . . (voice drags off).

Nurse: I didn't hear the end. I must not have been listening.

Rationalization: (Because) I must not have been listening.

Transformation: Your voice dropped. How are you feeling? (Focused question)

Pitfall 15—Stumped Silence

A stumped silence occurs when the client and the nurse are both stuck. There is an uncomfortable feeling that nothing is going on, that the nurse is confused.

A general guide in the instance of stumped silence is to metacomment about the confusion. That is, the nurse can comment about being confused, which can then lead to the client's focusing on her or his own confusion.

Examples of appropriate comments to break a stumped silence are:

- I'm having trouble figuring out what we do next. How are you feeling?
- At times it's hard to know exactly what to say. Let's see if we can continue in a few seconds.

Another option is to metacomment and briefly summarize what took place:

- I'm not sure where to go. Let's see, we were talking about ____ , you said ____ , and I said ____ just before we stopped. Do you have anything to add?

Pitfall 16—"Why" Questions

One of the great temptations when a client says virtually anything is to respond "Why did you say that?" The problem with "why" questions is that they imply that clients should come up with the underlying motivation of their actions or feelings, which is not what the nurse usually wants. In addition, many clients will feel that the nurse knows why and is testing them. They then get into guessing what the nurse thinks rather than examining their own motivation. "Why" questions can also easily be asked or perceived as accusatory. For example:

- Why do you feel that way?
- Why is the bandage off?
- Why were you late?

Almost any question can be rephrased as a less accusatory and more accurate statement. In the first of the examples given above, the nurse may really be asking for more information about the client's thoughts. A more accurate question would be, "What are some of the thoughts behind that feeling?" or more simply, "Tell me more about it." The second example could have been rephrased: "What happened to the bandage?" And the third could have been stated as, "You were late. What happened?" As a general guide, avoid "why" questions when interviewing clients.

EXERCISE IN TRANSFORMING WHY QUESTIONS

Change each of the following "why" questions on the left side of the page to another statement that gets to the same information. Suggested answers are given on the right of the page. Cover them until you have answered.

Why Question	Transformation
Why didn't you take your medication?	You didn't take your medication. What happened?
Why do you feel anxious?	Tell me more about your anxious- ness.
ious-	
Why are you depressed?	What's been going on?
Why do you think the clinic's bad?	What has happened to make you think the clinic's bad?

Why Question	Transformation
Why didn't you tell the doctor what you felt?	What prevented you from talking to the doctor?
Why aren't you happy about your new baby?	Tell me more about it.

INTEGRATING THE SKILLS WITH AVOIDANCE OF PITFALLS—AN EXERCISE

The following script of an interview has many examples of therapeutic and information-gathering skills, as well as a good number of pitfalls. As you read the script, identify each skill or strategy. When you find a pitfall, think about how it could be changed to promote increased self-regard and clearer communication.

A set of categorizations is provided with transformations of pitfalls on the right side of the page. Cover them until you have made your own choices. You may also want to use this method of interview analysis for analyzing role playing and taped interviews with clients. With practice, you will become adept at identifying your strengths and weaknesses as an interviewer and will, hopefully, attempt to correct ineffective techniques.

The Interview

The client, Mrs. C., is a home-bound senior citizen. She has arthritis, is recovering from a broken hip, and uses a walker. The purpose of the interview is a regularly scheduled check on her living situation and morale.

	Response Type
Nurse (Pulls chair over so the two are 3 feet apart and sitting):	Attends to seating
Hello Mrs. C., how have you been for the last week?	Open-ended question
Mrs. C.: So-so. You know. (Sighs)	Shares discrepancy, focused question on feelings
Nurse: You sighed just then, but said "so-so." How are you feeling?	
Mrs. C.: I don't know, I just don't have any energy.	
Nurse: You have no energy?	Probes
Mrs. C.: I just seem tired today.	
Nurse: Don't worry. It's probably the time of day. What did you do last week?	False reassurance, inappropriate change of topic. Transformation: You look tired. What's going on?

	Response Type
Mrs. C.: Well, I saw you on Tuesday. Wednesday I didn't do much at all, just watched TV.	
Nurse: Um-hmm.	Nonverbal reassurance
Mrs. C.: Thursday that lady, the physical therapist, came. She made me do all these exercises. (Laughs) I thought I was in the gym.	
Nurse: Does she work you too hard or have you do difficult things?	Multiple question. Transformation: What does she have you do?
Mrs. C.: I don't know. I've never seen anyone do the things the way she does them.	
Nurse (Waits silently)	Use of silence
Mrs. C.: How long will she be coming to see me. Why does she even bother?	
Nurse: How do you mean "why does she bother?"	Probe, request for clarification
Mrs. C.: It's just that. (Sighs) I don't know, I just think I'm never going to (starts to cry, voice softens) get better. I'm so embarrassed.	
Nurse: There, there, you'll feel better in a while. (Waits)	False reassurance. Transformation: It's OK to cry. Use of silence
Mrs. C. (Continues to cry, stops. Neither speaks, both look uncomfortable)	Stumped silence
Nurse: Tell me, Mrs. Clark, what were you thinking just now?	Probe
Mrs. C.: I was thinking about how I used to go to the community center before I fell. It was very nice there.	
Nurse (Nods head)	Nonverbal reassurance
Mrs. C.: I was just wondering what they were doing there this week.	
Nurse: You'd like to be able to find out what's going on?	Paraphrases
Mrs. C.: Um-hmm. I miss it. I have all of my friends there. There was even a special gentleman friend.	
Nurse: What was your relationship like with him?	Lead-in to "personal" area

Response Type

Mrs. C.: We used to see each other a lot. He'd even come and visit me here on weekends.

Nurse: Did you have meals here together?

Mrs. C.: Yes, occasionally.

Nurse: Did he visit every weekend? | Starts to use too many closed-ended questions. Transformation: Tell me about your relationship with the gentleman.

Nurse: Have you seen him since you were in the hospital?

Mrs. C.: Only once.

Nurse: Why hasn't he come? | Why question. Transformation: What do you think his reasons are for not coming?

Mrs. C.: I don't know.

Nurse: Well, I think you should call the center and find out. | Advice giving. Transformation: Have you considered calling to find out if he's OK?

Mrs. C.: No, I couldn't do that.

Nurse: OK, it was just a suggestion. | Defensiveness. Transformation: Um-hmm.

Mrs. C.: I just don't know what to do.

Nurse: About what? | Probe, Clarification

Mrs. C.: Can you really help me?

Nurse: I'll try my best. | Reassurance

Mrs. C.: Well, we were—we had been talking about living together like man and wife, but without getting married.

Nurse: You mean you'd do that without getting married? | Moralizing, Judging Transformation: What would prompt that choice?

Mrs. C.: We'd have to. Our social security checks would be cut if we were married. We can barely get by on the two checks as they are now.

Nurse: I see, you need both checks to get by. | Paraphrases

Mrs. C.: Right, only I haven't heard from him and I'm very worried.

Nurse: Is there anything I could do? | Focused question

Mrs. C.: Could you call the center and

Response Type

see if he's OK? I just can't bring
myself to do it.

Nurse: Sure. I'll let you know in 2 days
what I find out. Other than this, how
is everything else?

Mrs. C.: Fine, I can't complain. I take
my blood pressure pills. The
arthritis bothers me a little bit, but
no more than it usually does.

Nurse: Good, I'm glad to hear it. Let   Reassurance
me he sure I have everything
straight before I go. Everything is
going along OK as far as your
recovery goes. You're working
with the physical therapist. You're
taking your blood pressure pills.
Your arthritis bothers you a little,
but no more than usual. Your main
concern is your gentleman friend.
You haven't seen him and would   Summarizes, Closes
like me to call the center to find out
if he's OK. I'll get back to you in
2 days with the information.
Did I leave anything out?   Gives the client a chance to add
                                   information

Mrs. C.: No, but there is something
important I should add.

Nurse: What's that?   Probe

Mrs. C.: His name. I don't want you to
be bringing the wrong man around
here to move in with me! (Both laugh)

CONCLUSION

The first section of this book, Chapters 1 to 5, has presented content on
communication models, communication channels, communication styles,
therapeutic communication skills and information gathering skills and pitfalls. All these concepts and skills can be used in varying role relationships
and in different nursing contexts. Role relationships between nurses and
clients and between nurses and other health professionals are the focus of the
next section of this book (Chapters 6 to 8).

REFERENCES

Brammer, L. M. *The helping relationship: Process and skills,* (4th ed.). Englewood Cliffs, N.J.: Prentice-Hall, 1988.

Enelow, A. J., & Swisher, S. N. *Interviewing and patient care,* (3rd ed.). New York: Oxford University Press, 1986,

Rogers, C. R. *Client centered therapy.* Boston: Houghton Mifflin, 1951.

Satir, V. *The new peoplemaking.* Palo Alto, Calif.: Science and Behavior Books, 1988.

Yura, H., & Walsh, M. B. *The nursing process,* (4th ed.). Norwalk, Conn.: Appleton-Century-Crofts, 1987.

	# Communication
Section II	# and Role
	# Relationships

The nursing process is interactional. It represents a series of verbal and nonverbal behaviors that are goal directed (King, 1981). This section of the book focuses on communication dyads that represent interactions between two persons, one of whom is the nurse. A dyad is the basic unit of all communication interactions, with both persons in the dyad simultaneously interacting as senders and message receivers.

As we have seen in the first section of this book, dyadic communication can vary depending on the context, content, style, and channels used to convey messages. Nurses do not work in isolation; rather, they are part of a vast network of health workers representing different fields and interacting with each other. Figure II–1 illustrates this point.

Effective communication can be a challenge for nurses, as each health professional in this vast network may use and expect others to use a different set of communication skills. For example, how nurses interact with clients may be quite different from the way they interact with a dietitian. Also, the nurse is not the same person in the eyes of the dietitian that the same nurse is in the eyes of a peer, or a physician, or the client's family. How the two persons in the dyad "relate" to each other is the central concern; this relationship is so important it can determine the outcome of interactions regardless of verbal content, such as in the case of a nurse who is so busy and upset with an aide that he or she will ignore whatever the aide says.

Watzlawick's axiom IV presented in the first chapter bears repeating: "All communication relationships are either symmetrical or complementary, depending on whether they are based on equality or inequality" (1967, p. 70).

Symmetrical Relationships

Symmetrical relationships are based on equality; the partners tend to mirror each other's behavior (Watzlawick et al., 1967). That is, symmetrical

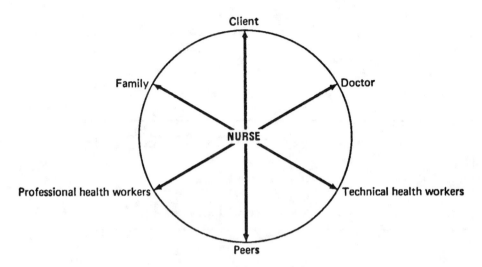

Figure II–1. Nurses' interactions.

relationships express or exchange the same basic communication behaviors: two friends talking about school, two clients sharing information about their surgery, or two staff nurses discussing their work in the hospital are examples of symmetrical relationships. In healthy symmetrical relationships, the partners can demonstrate a willingness to share feelings or give and accept constructive criticism.

Complementary Relationships

Complementary relationships are based on inequality; one partner assumes a superior or "one-up" position in the relationship (Watzlawick et al., 1967). Examples of complementary relationships can be parent–child, teacher–student, or nurse–client. Complementary relationships are not necessarily unhealthy or "bad" relationships. There are situations in which this type of communication relationship is necessary—for example, in the case of an acutely ill client and a nurse who is caring for this client. The ill client is dependent on the nurse, who is the decision maker for the care that is to be administered to the client.

Similarly, symmetrical relationships are not always "good" or normal relationships. Unhealthy symmetrical relationships can be characterized by competitiveness and lead to escalating, unstable relationships in which the partners fight and quarrel (Watzlawick et al., 1967).

The key point here is that nurses can learn to communicate effectively with others (clients and coworkers) using both symmetrical and complementary communication patterns. Some interactions call for symmetrical relationships and others for the complementary relationship, depending on the social or cultural context. Complementary and symmetrical communication patterns can even exist within the same relationship.

For example, two nurses (A and B) work in a geriatric extended-care facility. Nurse A asks nurse B to help her with one of A's assigned clients (complementary). Nurse A is instructing nurse B how to help her in this situation. Later at lunch, nurse A and nurse B exchange information about the client (symmetrical). In the afternoon, the head nurse shares some information about the client with nurse B. Nurse B relays this information to nurse A (complementary with nurse B one-up). Relationships that alternate between symmetrical and complementary patterns such as in the example of the two nurses just presented tend to be healthy relationships; this is to say, these changes from one pattern to the other (complementary to symmetrical or symmetrical to complementary) can be thought of as "homeostatic" (Watzlawick et al., 1967). In other words, nurses relate to others in symmetrical and complementary relationships depending on many different factors and influences.

Communication conflicts arise when patterns of symmetry and complementarity are used in unhealthy ways. For example, professionals who perceive themselves in relation to another as one-up (complementary) can use a defensive behavior such as blaming; other health professionals who perceive themselves as one-down (complementary) can use defensive behavior such as placating. Another area where communication conflicts arise is when both partners do not agree as to who is subordinate, superior, or equal to whom. In other words, one partner acts as if the other partner were equal, while at the same time the other partner assumes a complementary relationship exists!

This issue of symmetry–complementarity is an important one for nurses as they communicate with clients and other health care workers in different health settings. Again, it should be emphasized that both communication

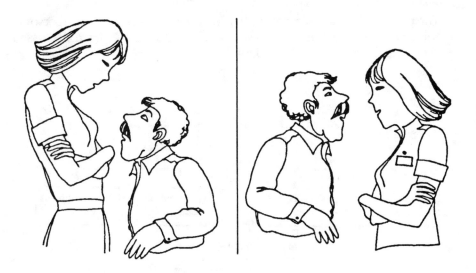

patterns can be mutually supportive and can be used constructively for the partners involved in the relationship.

An examination of the types of role relationships that are present within the health care delivery system helps us to develop greater clarity about our expectations of others, as well as the confusing set of expectations others have of us. These role relationships between nurses and other persons in the health care system are presented in Section II. The dyads will be discussed under three major groupings: nurse–nurse in Chapter 6; nurse–client in Chapter 7; and nurse–coworker (including physician) in Chapter 8. While it is recognized that other nurses are, strictly speaking, also coworkers in the health care system, a separate chapter has been devoted to the nurse–nurse dyadic relationships because of the unique problems that exist among nurses.

In addition to King and Watzlawick, two other theorists, Bakker, a physician, and Bakker-Rabdau, a nurse, have developed a conceptual framework of territoriality which is included in this second section. All persons have a sense of territoriality. Territory exists everywhere and can represent a concrete area of space with visible boundaries or an abstract concept with invisible boundaries. The Bakkers (1973) have provided a territorial model that we believe is most useful for nurses as they interact with others. The basic model (Figure II–2) portrays the four components under two domains, a private and a public one.

The public domain includes a person's interpersonal territory over which he or she has expertise or control and is divided into two areas: *psychological space*—the total amount of influence which one person exerts over the thoughts and feelings of others; and *action territory*—the area in which persons consider it their prerogative to act, exert control, make decisions, exercise their expertise, and take responsibility (i.e., an area of action which persons claim as their own). Much of our interactions in the work arena can be thought of as taking place in the action territory domain and are influenced by psychological space.

The private domain of territoriality includes two areas of intrapersonal territory; *privacy retreat* and *personal space*. These two areas are discussed further in the third section of this book.

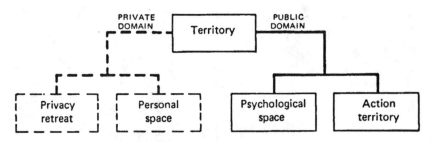

Figure II–2. Territorial model.

This section devotes separate chapters to nurse–nurse, nurse–client, and nurse–coworker communication. While communication skills and questions remain somewhat consistent across all the communication dyads, there are issues about relationships and context in each dyadic set that are unique, and make this discussion worthwhile for the nurse.

REFERENCES

Bakker, C. B., & Bakker-Rabdau, M. K. *No trespassing! Explorations in human territoriality*. San Francisco: Chandler & Sharp, 1973.

King, I. *A theory of nursing*. New York: Wiley, 1981.

Watzlawick, P., Beavin, J., & Jackson, D. *Pragmatics of human communication: A study of interactional patterns, pathologies and paradoxes*. New York: Norton, 1967.

6 Nurse–Nurse Dyads

BEHAVIORAL OBJECTIVES

By reading this chapter and participating in the exercises, students will be able to:

1. Understand the relationship of self-concept to one's nursing role behavior
2. Differentiate between personal and professional role identity
3. Describe the basic components of Bakkers' territoriality model
4. Understand the concepts of assertion and aggression as they interact in health care setting
5. Identify three components of stress

Communication is experienced individually. That is, we all have individual experiences and ways of categorizing our experience to understand the world (King, 1981). All of our professional communication is also influenced by our individuality. Issues that relate to how we view ourselves as individuals and professionals can have tremendous impact on our communication in the role of nurse. The first section of this chapter addresses nurses' individuality. Self-concept and self-awareness as they relate to personal and professional role identities are presented. The next section introduces the concept of territoriality and the use of assertion as a way to deal with stress and conflict when nurses interact with other nursing peers. The last section of the chapter presents some ideas about student nurses and several identified stressors which confront them in the clinical area.

SELF-CONCEPT AND SELF-AWARENESS

Self-Concept
Self-concept focuses on how we define and value ourselves. As we develop insight into ourselves as persons, we find it easier to relate to others (Hames & Joseph, 1986). Our self-concept develops throughout life as a result of our incorporating how others feel about us, as well as how others react to us. The

term "others" includes two important groups—*significant others* and *reference groups* (Brooks, 1985).

Significant others is a term that refers to individuals who exert a major influence on our lives. It includes members of our nuclear and extended family, as well as friends, teachers, and people in the community who have personal impact on us as individuals. Significant others influence our sense of self-concept in relation to many aspects of living, including values, matters of personal taste, and professional decisions, even though we may not be aware of this influence. They also influence self-concept through evaluations of work, performance, or action.

The second group subsumed under the term "others" is *reference groups*, those groups in which one has membership or wants to join. These groups can be either formal or informal. For example, in school, one joins clubs or teams; one can also be a member of the nursing profession and perhaps a study group, an art or music club, or a group of friends that socializes together. Each group has its own values, attitudes, and behaviors. By being a member, one can take on the same values and attitudes and behaviors as the group.

At the same time, if one's sense of self-concept is determined primarily or solely by reference group judgments, there would be no sense of personal value and almost a loss of individuality. It is possible to maintain a positive sense of self-worth in the light of negative evaluations in school or on the job without taking away from the validity of criticism or concerns about performance. In examining our self-concept and feelings, it is also important to assess the degree to which both significant others and reference groups influence self-worth.

It is important for nurses to have a positive self-concept, to "feel good about themselves" in order "to feel good about others." The authors' experience however, working with nurses in both hospital and community settings suggests that, too often, nurses do not pay enough attention to feeling good about themselves. Reasons for this can be attributed to the many demands made upon nurses in their professional roles resulting in added stress. Ways to address these problems are suggested later in this chapter.

Closely related to one's self-concept is one's sense of awareness of self and values. Self-awareness focuses on how cognizant persons are both of themselves in relation to others and their own self-concept. They must be able to answer such questions as: Who am I? What is important to me? and, Why do I want to be a nurse? (Brammer, 1988).

Self-awareness

Self-awareness focuses on how cognizant persons are both of themselves in relation to others and their own self-concept. Thus, self-awareness can include the individual's conscious understanding of her or his own feelings, how feelings are handled, limitations and strengths, the degree to which one feels validated by others, and the degree to which one realizes that he or she has choices in reacting to the environment, to others, and even to one's thoughts and reactions (Edinberg, 1985).

Self-awareness is a continuing part of our growth as individuals and professionals. It is also the first step in understanding how we interact with others or, as we put it in this book, the first step in understanding communication dyads. To know ourselves, each of us must understand our unique way of looking at others, as well as how others look at us. We react differently to similar experiences, because each of us has a unique system of beliefs and attitudes that determines our identity and its related self-concept.

PERSONAL AND PROFESSIONAL ROLE IDENTITIES

How can nurses answer the question regarding who they are and achieve a greater sense of self-awareness? One way is to become cognizant of one's personal self or identity in relation to one's professional self or identity. Although we may act differently in the work setting than in other situations, there does not have to be a distinct separation between these two identities in the work situation. The nurse ideally interacts with clients as an integrated self. For the purpose of providing further clarification of self-concept, however, these two identities have been separated.

Personal Identity
If one thinks about what one really has become since beginning a career in nursing, it might well be agreed that two identities, personal and professional, have emerged. One's personal identity includes one's emotional style, as well as the norms and values shaped by the family, schooling, religion, and friends. It is what makes one unique and different from others. Personal identity includes feelings, expectations, life experiences, sense of physical self (body image), knowledge, and sense of self-worth. Communication in health-care settings related to one's personal identity is usually on a horizontal or peer level.

Professional Identity
Professional identity encompasses characteristics that relate to the nursing profession. One shares these characteristics with other nurses, as well as common beliefs about nursing and one's role within the system of nursing. One also can be identified as a professional by one's way of dressing (uniform or lab coat), which serves as a visible sign of professional group identification. Communication in health-care settings, related to one's professional identity is usually on a vertical (one-up or one-down) level. Kelly (1985, p. 676) defines characteristics of a profession as follows:

- Specialized competence having an intellectual component
- Extensive autonomy in exercising this special competence

- Strong commitment to a career based on a special competence
- Influence and responsibility in the use of special competence
- Development of training facilities that are controlled by the professional group
- Decision making governed by internalized standards

An important issue for nursing is whether nurses as professionals fulfill the above criteria compared with other professions. Most nursing leaders think that nursing has attained the status of a profession. Yet others have stated that nursing is only *in the process of becoming* a profession and has not reached the status of full professional maturity.

Review the criteria which are presented in the preceding paragraphs once again. Weigh each criterion carefully and then ask yourself the following questions:

- Are nurses' behaviors and actions professional in relation to the criteria?
- Is nursing *more* or *less* professional than medicine, the law, or engineering?
- Do you see any problems in becoming "overprofessionalized"?

As nurses gain experience in the health-care setting, they often experience a shift from a personal role identity to a professional role identity. The most experienced nurses often have learned to integrate both identities, thus maintaining their personal warmth as individuals and administering competent care to clients.

EXERCISE IN PERSONAL VERSUS PROFESSIONAL ROLE IDENTITY

1. Break up into pairs.
2. Look at the following list of statements in Column 1 (personal identity) and Column 2 (professional identity) and rate yourselves [using a scale of 1 (low) to 5 (high)] on your attitude about yourself in reference to each statement:

Column 1 (Personal Identity)	Column 2 (Professional Identity)
I am usually happy.	I have a strong desire to help others.
What others think about me doesn't affect me.	I like new experiences.
I am easy-going.	I like all types of people.
I have lots of patience.	I find satisfaction in hard work.
I am open and sincere.	I like to feel needed.
I have high expectations.	I am committed to my chosen career.

3. Discuss the similarities and dissimilarities between yourself and your partner with reference to each column. Did you find more or less mutual agreement with the statements in Column 1 or Column 2?

4. Discuss the following: When do personal and professional identities clash? When do they fit together? What kinds of communication occur in each case?

ASSERTION/AGGRESSION IN NURSING

There is no question that assertion skills are a necessary part of nurses' communication repertoire in today's society. Nurses need to be able to be assertive, that is, clearly defend their rights and express their wants to clients, as well as coworkers and superiors in a variety of settings. Responding assertively is also a way of enhancing one's self-esteem.

Assertion training was initially introduced in the late 1960s as a therapeutic tool for psychiatric patients who were considered passive (Edinberg, 1975). Others, mainly women's groups, were quick to adopt assertion as a way of helping individuals cope with feelings of inadequacy and inferiority. Virtually all nursing schools have introduced some sort of assertion component into their curriculum, in part to provide nurses with appropriate alternatives to traditional passive role of the nurse. Assertive behavior, in the traditional sense, is that type of interpersonal behavior that enables individuals to act in their own best interest, to stand up for themselves without anxiety, and to exercise their rights without denying those of others (Bond, 1988). It is a direct, honest, and appropriate expression of one's feelings, opinions, and beliefs and implies taking responsibility of one's actions.

Passive behavior, in the traditional sense, is interpersonal behavior that allows the individual's rights to be violated in one of two ways: (a) the person violates her or his own right by ignoring them, or (b) the person permits others to infringe on his or her rights. Passive behavior pays off by enabling the individual to avoid potentially unpleasant conflicts with others; however, various unpleasant internal consequences—hurt feelings and lower self-esteem—are then likely (Bond, 1988).

Finally, aggressive behavior is interpersonal behavior in which a person stands up for his or her rights in such a way that the rights of the other person are violated. Aggressive behavior dominates, humiliates, or "puts the other person down" as opposed simply to expressing one's honest emotions or thoughts (Bond, 1988). Aggressive behavior is reactive, unplanned behavior.

In the past, nurses were taught to be acquiescent, passive, and submissive in their relationships with other people in the course of their work. Passive, nonassertive nurses possessed those qualities most valued by others within the profession, as well as by those outside of it.

We have little quarrel with the benefits of respecting the rights of others and being nonblaming in communication style, but it appears that, even with an assertive stance, certain requests, needs, or statements, by their nature, have to be seen as "aggressive" in that they seek to take resources from another person (Bakker & Bakker-Rabdau, 1973). As an alternative, Bakkers' model of territoriality emphasizes the relative merits of assertion and aggression in the development of one's "territory" and relationships with others in the health care setting. This model can readily be applied to nurses as well as any group of workers.

BAKKERS' MODEL OF TERRITORIALITY

How would you respond in the following situation?

> You are the evening charge nurse and for the third night in a row, the night nurse who is to relieve you is about 15 minutes late.

Do you ignore this and say nothing? Do you express your anger at his or her behavior? Do you use your assertion skills and state that you would like him or her to be on time in the future?

This vignette is particularly important because it raises questions of *territoriality* (Bakker & Bakker-Rabdau, 1973). Territoriality can be thought of as the need for and processes connected with obtaining "territory" (resources, responsibilities, power, or ability to control others' behavior). It is relevant in all relationships between nurses as well as with others within the health care setting, including clients and physicians.

Territoriality has been defined as the behavior used to defend "turf" and as an innate drive. Some theories based on studies with animals as well as humans have proposed that territoriality satisfies certain basic needs, such as security and identity (Mallon-Palmer, 1980; King, 1981; Shaw, 1983; Clark, 1984). Other theorists make the assumption that territoriality is not only an innate drive in persons, but much of the behavior can be *learned* as one socializes with others (Bakker & Bakker-Rabdau, 1973; Lazarus, 1973; Bakker, Bakker-Rabdau, & Breit, 1978; Hernandez & Mauger, 1980).

The Management of Territory

Managing or acquiring new territory requires the use of two types of behavioral skills—assertiveness and aggressiveness. Bakkers' territoriality model is basically one of ownership; you own or you do not own. If you own, you can assert; if you do not own but want to own, then you need to aggress to obtain the territory you desire. Aggression is not "bad" or negative behavior. In fact, it is appropriate and necessary in many instances.

In this framework, there are many ways to be aggressive, all of which are congruent behavior. There are instances, however, when you are in a one-down relationship or do not have a right to some control over the resources, but you still choose to aggress or expand your territory. The act of taking charge, gaining control, or making your viewpoint known in this instance may be perceived to be transgressive. Transgression means taking away one's territory without permission.

A final point in this discussion is that the territory which is the object of ownership includes physical or geographic territory (such as actual possessions or space for an office) and/or abstract or psychological territory (such as ideas, rights, privileges). Consider the following situation:

> Two nurses, Abby and Betty, work in the same unit. At lunch Betty asks Abby if she would be willing to work on Saturday (Abby's day off), as she (Betty) would like to attend a wedding. Abby responds that she does not wish to work on her day off, as she has made plans for the weekend.

In this situation, Betty is "aggressing" on Abby's territory. That is, by asking a favor of Abby, Betty is attempting to expand her territory. She desires to go to a wedding, see old friends, and possibly meet some new ones. Abby, on the other hand, is asserting; she is defending her territory, and responds by telling Betty "No." In any life situation people can either defend (using assertiveness) their territory or expand it (using aggressiveness).

The success and value of aggression depends on how one uses the aggressive act (or one's ability to use "aggressiveness" skills), the attractiveness of the territory to be acquired, and the hope of acquiring that territory. To aggress properly, one must be constantly aware that wanting a territory does not give one rights to the territory. Ownership bestows rights, including the right to defend the territory. In this framework, aggression is indicative of *growth* and *exploration*, rather than destruction, and is accompanied with experiencing new areas and a sense of adventure. Thus aggression can be viewed as potentially positive behavior. Its appropriateness and value should be considered carefully by nurses, who work in an age of expanding territory in terms of responsibilities and knowledge about care of our clients.

Assertion and Aggression as They Interact in the Health Setting

In a dyadic interaction, as one person's territory is expanded, the other's is reduced. When one's territory is "invaded" by another, the appropriate response is assertiveness. A "territorial defense" should be direct and specific to retain or regain control over the intruded upon area.

Look again at the situation involving Abby and Betty. Abby could have granted Betty her request and worked on her scheduled day off, but really not wanting to. She would then have *failed to assert*, with a subsequent reaction of hostility. Hostility often ends up being destructive energy used to injure the aggressor. Abby, in this case, would have been angry; she would have felt Betty has taken advantage of her. Rather than confronting Betty directly about her anger (an assertive response), Abby perhaps would choose to tell Connie, another nurse in the unit about the situation. Connie would be brought into the interaction and can be counted on to give advice such as "You should not have covered for her." Connie may well harbor some resentment about Betty as well.

Interactions such as this one are common. Think of it again in terms of your own behavior. How often do you choose to not defend your territory when it is "attacked"? It is worth considering if your reluctance to do so comes from realistic expectations about the others (some people are not very open to assertive responses from nurses or coworkers), expectations about yourself (it can be quite difficult for some people to be assertive with superiors), or expectations about the nature of the situation (in some situations, nurses do not own the territory, in others they own a lot of territory). Finally, even with these considerations, it is frequently worthwhile deciding the positive and negative outcomes of failing to be assertive when your territory is invaded by others.

EXERCISE IN EXAMINING ASSERTION VERSUS AGGRESSION

Examine the following situations. Identify the territory as well as the owner of the territory. Then look at the responses to the situations. Which are assertive in that they defend existing territory? Which are aggressive in that they seek to acquire more territory?

1. You are the charge nurse. You come into a client's room in a hospital and find that he or she has not received his or her medication. You point out the problem to the responsible nurse.
2. The ostomy nurse in your hospital asks you to leave the floor to meet a visitor in the lobby when you are the only registered person on duty. You say, politely, "No, I cannot do this."
3. You are on a team of nurses and want to take charge of one of the new clients on the floor. You make your request to the group in a team meeting.
4. You go to your supervisor and gently remind her that you have been working extra hours, have the best attendance record on the shift, and, although it's your fault you have never made this known and you could understand it if she said "no," but you would like to have a raise to pay your rent.

> Discuss these four situations: the first two are assertive situations
> and the last two are aggressive situations. What are the benefits when
> you assert and when you aggress in each of the four situations?

Action Territory

One type of territory is *action territory* which is directly related to the nurses'
roles in the work environment. This is defined as ". . . the area in which a
person considers it his or her prerogative to act, exert control, make decisions, exercise one's expertise, and take responsibility, in other words an area
of action which a person claims as his or her own" (Bakker & Bakker-Rabdau,
1973). Action territory includes the functions one performs, his or her rights
and privileges, and the status which one attributes to one's professional
nursing role.

EXERCISE IN PUBLIC DOMAIN—ACTION TERRITORY
WITH ASSERTION/AGGRESSION RESPONSES
IN SITUATIONS

For each of the following situations, define the person who owns the
territory, and then determine if the response was assertive or aggressive. Compare these responses with what your own response would
have been in the same situation.

1. You are assigned to give medications on your unit. When you return from a coffee break, you find that another nurse has taken on
   the job without informing you in order to help you out. You tell her
   that you were assigned to give the medications and it is your job.
2. The nurse manager in charge of the unit where you are working as
   a "prn" nurse assigns you to care for a client who has specific
   nursing needs related to an area in which you have no experience.
   You inform the nurse manager of this fact.
3. You are assigned to several difficult clients for the day and notice
   your colleague has an easy assignment. You ask her to help you
   out.

In situation 1, the action territory of passing out the medications for the
unit was yours. The other nurse aggressed on your territory by taking on the
job without asking you. Your response in defending your territory was an
assertive one.

In situation 2, the nurse manager requested you to care for a particular
client. When you told him or her that you had no experience with this type of
client, your response was an *assertive* response.

In situation 3, your territory was the heavy assignment. You attempted to aggress on your colleague by asking her to help you out. Your response, therefore, was an *aggressive* one. If your colleague told you "no," she or he asserted; if she or he said "yes," she or he did not assert and therefore lost some of her or his territory.

In the work world, it is not enough to consider how to obtain territory. Realistically, once territory is obtained, it must be managed. Your skill in managing the boundaries and areas of your action territory will depend on your knowledge of your work tasks, responsibilities, the "system" in which you work, and, of course, your communication skills discussed in this book.

Territories can be managed in three ways—decreasing the size of the territory, attaining additional skills, and obtaining help from others (situation 3). Each of these management areas may have "aggressive" acts as part of its successful management. Each has "assertive" components, as well.

The use of assertion and aggression skills helps nurses to handle and even prevent stress and conflict in the health care setting. As you read the following sections on stress and conflict, think about how you might use assertion and aggression skills to either prevent or resolve some of the problems that arise.

STRESS

Stress is an expected part of any relationship. An understanding of the causes of stress, of how people cope with it, and of the resulting communication barriers is also beneficial.

In the hospital, clients are ill, in pain, or helpless. In the community setting, clients are often poor and have many unfulfilled needs. Nurses work with atypical populations, namely, sick individuals. As a result, they can feel a sense of helplessness and stress. The term "stress" means many different things to different people (Humphrey, 1988). It has been used to describe the events that trigger a "stressful" response, the physiological reactions to stress-invoking events (such as rapid heart beat, perspiring, elevated blood pressure, and unsettled feelings in the stomach), and behavioral reactions to the events and physiological responses to them (such as overeating, driving too fast, taking too much alcohol or other drugs).

Three important components to stress are: the stress-inducing event (stimulus), a perception by the individual that the event is threatening to self-esteem, and the physiological and behavioral responses to stress (response).

Stress-producing events vary for nurses in their working settings. The following work-related stressors, however, have been most often identified: patients, understaffing, administration, coworkers, time, physicians, supplies and equipment, and compensation. The most frequent effective coping mechanism identified by nurses is "talking things over with others" either with a colleague or family member (Humphrey, 1988). Making use of significant others and using effective communication skills can help to decrease or eliminate unhealthy physiological and behavioral reactions to stress-invoking events.

Donnelly (1980) refers to two ways of dealing with stress: reactive and active. In reacting to stress, one experiences the fight-or-flight syndrome as the only recourse. One chooses to fight the stressful situation through the use of aggression or by using defensive behaviors ("it's not my fault"). One copes with this stress by turning it inward and finding satisfaction in other ways: eating, drinking, smoking, sleeping, or becoming depressed (Scully, 1980). Active ways of dealing with stress are, first, to identify the *signs* of stress and then to locate the *sources*, some of which can be managed through the use of assertion. Having done this, one can learn to control his or her behavior through the utilization of exercises or relaxation techniques. Maintaining a sense of personal worth despite defeats, tolerating or relieving the distressors, and maintaining rewarding or interpersonal relationships all help one to cope with the stressful situation (Jacobson & McGrath, 1983). Along with these general strategies, we also recommend specific programs, such as the self-modification behavior techniques and the relaxation response outlined in Humphrey's book, *Stress in the Nursing Profession* (1988).

CONFLICT

While some stressors are due to circumstances beyond anyone's control (such as having a deadline to file your income tax), one way to decrease stress is to handle conflicts that lead to stress situations. Conflict *always exists* when two or more interdependent parties interact. A certain degree of conflict is healthy; conflict can result in enhanced relationships; it allows one to grow and learn. On the other hand, too much conflict can be damaging to a relationship. One's aim is to arrive at some point between these two extremes. People approach conflict in five different ways (Lutjens, 1983; Marriner, 1982):

1. Avoid situations that provoke controversy or disagreement.
2. Smooth it over by false reassurance, thinking that everything will be OK.
3. Overpower it in an authoritarian manner.
4. Bargain and reach a compromise solution.
5. Identify the underlying causes and through understanding, work out a solution—the problem-solving approach.

While there are some "artful dodgers" (as in statement 1 above) who constantly avoid stress in order to survive, this is not a response that promotes psychological growth. Again, the "peacemakers" (statement 2) do not get at the heart of the problem. Statement 3, which on the surface appears to be a solution for conflict, does not probe at finding the reasons for the stress. Statement 4 represents one approach to a solution to the problem. In the resolution of the conflict, usually both sides have to give.

We are able to characterize how we tend to react to conflict by identifying with one of the above approaches. Identifying the reasons for the conflict and attempting to resolve the underlying causes (statement 5) is the most effective, collaborative approach in dealing with conflict situations. This approach is often referred to as a win-win situation. It also involves utilizing the problem-solving approach, and as previously stated, once the problem is identified, the resolution of the problem is not as difficult as it was before the problem was pinpointed.

When dealing with conflict there are two important points to keep in mind: (1) No one approach to conflict resolution is the best in every given situation. There are times when avoidance in the conflict situation is an acceptable communication behavior; and (2) nurses can change their approaches in order to adapt to the demands of a new situation.

When conflicts do occur, some nurses utilize defensive communication patterns in which they spend most of their time and energy defending themselves. Because they have perceived themselves as being threatened, they do not listen to others but concentrate on the impact of their behavior on others. It is possible to learn to anticipate these defensive behaviors and recognize the attacks are not directed toward one's self-worth, thus depersonalizing the conflict. The skills concerning use of channels, assertion, and empathy that have been presented in other sections of this book are helpful in conflict resolution.

NURSE–NURSE DYADS

Communication between staff nurses in the clinical area is *peer* communication and reflects a symmetrical relationship. Communication between the student nurse and staff nurse in the clinical area can vary from *peer* communication to *one-up/one-down* communication in which the student is in the subordinate position and the staff nurse assumes a superior position. This complementary communication between student and staff is seldom referred to in the literature. Since there is a likelihood that the majority of persons reading this book are students, it is worth discussing.

Common complementary relationships between nurses include leader–follower, helper–helpee, or clinical instructor–student. When a student is one member of the relationship, the nature of the relationship depends on the student's level of development and professionalization within the nursing program. In addition, how students perceive themselves and how the staff perceives the students in relation to expertise and experience can differ, thus creating communication problems:

Sue Taylor, a staff nurse on a surgical unit in a community hospital, places high priority on high-visibility tasks. She always makes sure that her clients' physical needs are met. When students are assigned to the floor, Sue works with them; she often conveys the attitude that they have much to learn. Also, Sue acts as if she doubts whether they could assume responsibility for client care without her direct supervision.

A beginning student, Cheryl Smith, is assigned to Sue's floor. Cheryl is to care for a colostomy client having daily irrigations. Cheryl had looked forward to having this experience and had studied about colostomy clients and their treatment before coming to the unit. Sue's comment to Cheryl, however, regarding the colostomy irrigation was:

"Oh, you're not ready to do that!"

Obviously Cheryl felt she was more capable of assuming responsibility in client care than Sue did. One action could be for Cheryl to consult with her clinical instructor; however if the clinical instructor is not immediately available, then Cheryl has to decide how to handle the difference of opinion with Sue, such as asking Sue to have a cup of coffee and telling her how she (Cheryl) feels.

Student and staff nurses often perceive the environment in which they are working differently. Students view the unit as "foreign" territory with no ownership rights; that is they are unfamiliar with the members of the system, and its communication patterns. The spontaneity and sense of equality that prevailed in the classroom or on campus is supplanted by a climate that is uncertain and controlled by others.

On the other hand, graduate nurses perceive their work environment as familiar territory; they know the routines and standard paper work. They wear the same uniform and speak the same caring and technical language. They have an established sense of trust in other nurses with whom they work.

Both staff and students alike find themselves on fixed time schedules. The following interaction was heard by one of the authors in a hospital setting. The student nurse was feeling anxious because she was behind in her assignment and for some unknown reason the clock on the unit was displaying incorrect time.

Student: What time is it?
Nurse: It's late. It is very late.
Student: What time is it?
Nurse: You must learn to use your time more efficiently! Hurry, it's late.
Student: What time is it?

It is difficult to say where this communication cycle began or ended, from the way the two were interacting; it could have taken them an eternity to find out what the actual time was. The nurse obviously was so anxious that the student was behind on her assignment, that she could not respond to the direct question.

We all live in the here (space) and now (time); therefore, time becomes valuable. In our role as nurses, it is always possible that we will not be able to finish assigned tasks within the time period afforded them. How nurses prioritize their time is an expression of their feelings about what is important to them. If a nurse is willing to spend time with a student, it is reasonable to assume that the nurse places a high value on the communication interaction. Some nurses become skilled in utilizing time spent in communication to good advantage. Others may assign students to low priority in their minds and not spend much time communicating with them.

Differences in perception of the hospital setting and in the concept of time, as well as the internal factors of self-worth and varying degrees in ability to perform nursing tasks, can lead to defensive communication between student and staff nurse. The result will be placating, blaming, super-reasonableness, and irrelevance—characteristics of closed communication.

Given the possibilities for closed communication—as well as ones for open communication that is efficient, congruent, and raises self-worth—how can the student learn to communicate effectively in the various clinical settings that are encountered? The usual answer is "through trial and error plus modeling the instructor." Also, the more congruent the response of the student, the more able he or she will be to pick up the accepted "style" of communication that fits the setting and to decide how to communicate on a sensible basis. The following exercise represents a step towards determining the components of effective student–nurse communication:

EXERCISE IN STUDENT–NURSE COMMUNICATION

1. Write or describe three situations in which you, as a student, were effective in communicating with a nurse. That is, the message sent was the message received, the message was congruent, or that self-worth was maintained on both sides.
2. Now, write or describe three situations in which your communication was ineffective with a nurse. That is, the message sent was *not* the one received.
3. For each of the three messages in Step 2 above, guess what "went wrong:"
   a. No understanding of other's words
   b. "Personality" (conflict of styles)
   c. Conflict of channels (e.g., one visual, one auditory)
   d. Time
   e. Stress
   f. Lack of trust

> **g.** Differences in perception of abilities
> **h.** Difference of opinion.
> **4.** In the large group, discuss how some of these could be rectified.

In addition to the territorial and time factors that influence student–nurse communication, there are three common difficulties that students encounter in communicating with nurses.

1. *High expectations.* Most students begin clinical experiences expecting to know all the answers, as well as to administer client care with little or no difficulty. These are unreal expectations.
2. *An inability to define the problem.* The most difficult step of the problem-solving model presented in Chapter 7 is pinpointing the problem. A pertinent question to ask is, "Who owns the problem?"
3. *The reluctance on the part of nurses to express feelings and emotions.* Many people hide their true feelings, that is, they tend to act differently from the way they feel. The environment in which nursing care is administered encourages the masking of real feelings. The concept of the "good nurse" leading to a professional bedside manner fosters a stereotype of a nonlistener who interacts with people on a superficial level.

CONCLUSION

This chapter examined several important concepts and skills for nurses in their work with each other as well as their work with clients and other health professionals. Both our sense of self-worth (self-image) and sensitivity to ourselves and how we interact with others (self-awareness) have tremendous impact on our communication with other nurses. In addition, we have to be prepared for the inevitability of stressful moments and conflicts in giving health care. Effective communication skills discussed in the previous section of this text are one set of tools. Assertion, stating what one needs or expects in a direct but unhostile manner, is another area for skill development. A third area is the use of "aggression" to obtain resources or a sense of territory necessary to function as a competent and professional nurse.

REFERENCES

Bakker, C. B., & Bakker-Rabdau, M. K. *No trespassing! Explorations in human territoriality.* San Francisco: Chandler & Sharp, 1973.
Bakker, C. B., Bakker-Rabdau, M. K., & Breit, S. The measurement of assertiveness

and aggressiveness. *Journal of Personality Assessment*, 1978, 42(3), 277–284.

Bond, M. Understanding assertiveness. *Nursing Times*, 1988, 84(9), 61–64.

Bond, M. Assertiveness discussion; Making your point. *Nursing Times*, 1988, 84(12), 73–76.

Brammer, L. *The helping relationship: Process and skills* (4th ed.). Englewood, N. J.: Prentice-Hall, 1988.

Brooks, W. *Speech communication* (5th ed.). Dubuque, Iowa: Wm. C. Brown, 1985.

Clark, D. K. *The relationship of assertiveness and aggressiveness with job satisfaction.* Master's thesis (unpublished), University of Illinois, 1984.

Donnelly, G. F. Why you just can't take it anymore! *RN*, May 1980, 34–37.

Edinberg, M. A. *Behavioral assessment and assertion training of the elderly.* Doctoral dissertation (unpublished) University of Cincinnati, 1975.

Edinberg, M. A. *Mental health practice with the elderly.* Englewood Cliffs, New Jersey: Prentice-Hall, 1985.

Hames, C. C. & Joseph, D. H. *Basic concepts of helpings: A holistic approach* (2nd ed.). Norwalk: Appleton-Century-Crofts, 1986.

Hernandez, S. K. & Mauger, P. A. Assertiveness, aggressiveness and Eysenchk's personality variables. *Personality and Individual Differences*, 1980, 1(2), 143–149.

Humphrey, J. *Stress in the nursing profession.* Springfield, Ill.: Charles C. Thomas, 1988.

Jacobson, S. F., & McGrath, H. M. (eds.) *Nurses under stress.* New York: John Wiley & Sons, 1983.

Kelly, L. Y. *Dimensions of professional nursing* (5th ed.). New York: MacMillan Publishing Co., 1985.

King, I. *A theory for nursing.* New York: Wiley, 1981.

Lazarus, A. On assertive behavior: A brief note. *Behavior Therapy*, 1973, 4, 697–699.

Lutjens, L. R. The name of this game is conflict. *Nursing Management*, 1983, 14(6) 23–24.

Mallon-Palmer, M. Personal space theories: Lessons for nurses. *The Australian Nurses' Journal*, 1980, 10(5), 36–38.

Marriner, A. Managing conflict. *Nursing management*, 1982, 13(6) 23–31.

Scully, R. Stress in the nurse. *American Journal of Nursing*, 1980, 80(5), 912–914.

Shaw, R. J. *Privacy and action territory in a nursing home population.* Master's thesis (unpublished), University of Illinois, 1983.

7 | Nurse–Client Dyads

BEHAVIORAL OBJECTIVES

By reading this chapter and participating in the exercises, students will be able to:

1. Describe how the changing roles of client and nurse have influenced the nurse–client relationship
2. Recognize the psychological and sociological aspects of illness
3. Discuss patterns of communication in nurse–client complementary relationships
4. Identify labeling: "hostile client," "good client," and "good nurse"
5. Understand the use of a problem-solving approach to help client to facilitate solutions relating to illness and/or health

Each nurse–client interaction is unique; it occurs only once; it can never recur in the same place at the same time. Nurse–client interactions differ from those in many other dyads in that they are purposeful. The two persons involved come together for a purpose—to set goals in order to help the client cope with human responses to actual or potential health problems. These goals are mutually set by the nurse and client; if they are achieved, a *transaction* has occurred (King, 1981).

A key factor in understanding nurse–client interactions is perception, or interpretation of the experience. Nurses perceive clients through a complex process of selecting, organizing, and constructing sensory data into their experiences. Thus, nurses and clients can interpret interactions differently, depending on their individual views and experiences. In other words, similar experiences with a client could communicate two totally different meanings to two different nurses.

One way in which the nurse or the client interact with each other is based upon their perception or view of themselves. Each person has a concept of self which he or she brings to the dyadic interaction.

Nurse–Client Relationship

If we ever stop to think about what we bring to the nurse–client relationship, the list would be long. Here are a few examples:

- Feelings
- Values
- Fears
- Motivations
- Prejudices
- Goals

Our unique make-up, our background, all the things that make us tick contribute to the nurse–client dyadic relationship. A knowledge of who we are, who we would like to be, how we think others see us, and what motivates our actions are all part of our own uniqueness. Such questions as "How well do you know yourself?" "How does this knowledge of yourself influence your perception of the client?" or "How does this knowledge influence the manner in which you decode and react to the client's message?" are often never answered. The relationships nurses have with clients are directly related to their perceptions of themselves, and to the congruence between one's own feelings and the facts. Confusion between one's own feelings and the facts can lead to ineffective communication. The following situation serves as an example:

> Mr. Stone, who was 87 years old, was getting progressively more disoriented. His wife, a nurse, had been caring for him in their home. When Mrs. Dixon, the visiting nurse, made a home visit to see how things were, Mrs. Stone, who had previously been able to cope, burst into tears, and stated that the time had come to place Mr. Stone in a nursing home. "He keeps saying that he wants to go home. He doesn't know me and I can no longer communicate with him. Yesterday I had to call the police because he ran outside and down the street in his bathrobe, looking for his home. I'll just have to place him in the nursing home where I have reserved a bed for him."
>
> Mrs. Dixon then remembered when her grandfather was placed in a nursing home by his daughter (Mrs. Dixon's mother). The grandfather was not disoriented and actually became confused after his admission. He died soon thereafter. Mrs. Dixon's internal response was, "I'd never do that to my parents!" And she recommended to Mrs. Stone that Mr. Stone not be placed in a nursing home.

Mrs. Dixon's use of her own emotional feelings was not helpful to Mrs. Stone, who needed support for what was a difficult and possibly correct decision. This is not to say, however, that the feelings should have been ignored. The underlying concerns about when to institutionalize a loved one could have been used by the visiting nurse to empathize with Mrs. Stone. It should also be noted that the visiting nurse gave advice (an interviewing pitfall) rather than working with Mrs. Stone to make her own decision and feel good about it.

The whole issue about *how* to use one's inner reactions is complicated. The more self-awareness, the more one is likely to match relevant parts of experience to current reality. Most people work on developing an increased sense of self-awareness throughout their lives. Increased knowledge comes through daily experiences interacting with all people, not just clients. Merely having the experience does not, however, mean that anyone, including nurses, automatically learns from what has transpired. Self-awareness is usually the result of active thinking about one's own interaction with others and consideration of both positive and negative feedback from others. It is through the process of experience and thinking and integrating it with knowledge that self-awareness emerges.

Radical changes in the health care delivery system have also influenced the nurse–client relationship. As a result, different communication patterns have emerged between the nurse and the client.

Look at the following incident which occurred to one of our colleagues:

J.C. was admitted to the hospital for a cholescystectomy. Her preoperative x-rays revealed a hiatal hernia which could be treated conservatively by diet, medications, and weight loss.

After gallbladder surgery and before her discharge, the student nurse who had been responsible for J.C.'s daytime care discussed the hiatal hernia with her, stating that she had read her textbook and telling J.C. what the recommended treatment was. Then the student nurse asked, "What do you think?" In addition, the student nurse would continually ask J.C. questions such as: "What do you know about this?", "Have you tried this?", "What worked for you?"

Before discharge from the hospital, J.C. was approached by a medical resident, whose comment regarding her hiatal hernia was: "If you do not follow the recommended diet and medication orders, you will have esophageal scarring and regurgitation which will necessitate painful dilation with a catheter."

Can you determine the difference in the two approaches? In the first, the student nurse attempted to involve the client in setting the goals for her health care and measuring the effectiveness of her interventions. Both client and nurse assumed active roles, whereas in the second, the physician played an active role while the client assumed a passive role. The physician assumed that the client would abide by instructions and cooperate in the carrying out of the treatment.

Historically, the nurse–client relationship centered around the nurse caring *for* and attending *to* the client in an environment of trust. The nurse *managed* the interaction between client and environment, often focusing on physical needs and emphasizing the qualities of nurturing, assistance, and succoring. The client's role was typically one of dependence and submissiveness.

Contrast this relationship with today's nurse–client relationship. It has been reformulated over time into an interactional process of negotiated decision making by two active participants (Artinian, 1983). Ideally, the relationship is characterized as *dynamic* in that the interaction influences the behaviors of each person (Armstrong, 1983). It is viewed as a "symbolic interactional process," the result of which is change and growth for both nurse and client (Kasch, 1984).

Client's Role

The term *role* implies a set of behaviors which others perceive as acceptable, related to a given situation (Brooks & Kleine-Kracht, 1983). The client's set of expected behaviors is not the same as it was a decade ago. Today's clients live in a society where they know more about disease than the average physician did at the turn of the century. Many clients expect the right to make their own health care decisions, and if they do not receive it, they will demand it.

The whole question of territoriality in the health care setting has shifted. No longer is one's body the property of health professionals in a hospital setting, but the body as well as all health information relating to it, have become part of the client's territory. Clients have a right to know their blood pressure readings, the laboratory results, and the x-ray interpretations. Inherent with this privilege is an adequate explanation to provide understanding of health or illness status. Today's clients:

- Question
- Assert
- Treat themselves
- Are involved in decision making

The self-help movement in health care is clearly related to the new roles clients are taking in their interaction with health professionals.

Self-Care. All persons have the innate ability to care for themselves. Self-care includes those activities that a person initiates or performs on his or her own behalf to health. It is characterized by the client acting as a peer or equal of the nurse in the setting of goals for his or her health.

Self-care programs have been incorporated within the structures of the hospitals themselves. In one such hospital, the incorporation of self-care education model included the following phases (Caporael-Katz, 1983):

- Provision of time for client expression of feelings of anger and frustration at the lack of care within the health care system
- Raising client self-esteem lowered due to presence of complementary relationships within the health care system

- Practice of self-care skills that could be applied immediately
- Presentation of alternative views of health issues
- Critical evaluation of both traditional medicine and alternative therapies

The benefits of this program in terms of positive client feedback, number of clients served, and attendance at multisession health education courses have been tremendous. In addition, while some nurses felt threatened with loss of power, other nurses felt "freed from playing interpersonal power games, withholding information and pretending to have the ultimate answers" (Caporael-Katz, 1983, p. 6).

Nurse's Role

A major purpose of nursing is to maximize the client's potential for self-care. Orem (1985) describes three nursing systems to meet client needs based on a self-care theoretical framework. Each of the three systems represents a variation in the roles of the nurse and client in the performance of health care activities required by the client. The first system, *wholly compensatory*, is one in which the client has no active role in his or her performance of care. The nurse's role is centered around doing for the client who is in a totally dependent state. There are three types of clients for whom *wholly compensatory* care is appropriate: clients who are (1) comatose, (2) unable to make rational decisions, and (3) aware and able to communicate, but are physically incapacitated.

The second system, *partially compensatory*, is one in which client and nurse perform care measures involving manipulative tasks or ambulation. The client is moving between dependent and independent states. The communication relationship is alternating between complementary and symmetrical patterns in which both the nurse and the client perceive themselves as equal. The balance in a partially compensatory nursing system, however, is toward a complementary relationship in which the nurse is superior to the client. In addition, five methods of helping—doing or acting for another, guiding or directing, providing physical support, providing psychological support, and providing an environment that supports development—may be in use at the same time.

The third system, *educative–supportive*, is one in which the client is able to perform measures of self-care but still needs nursing assistance, which can include combinations of any of the five methods of helping. This is the only system where the client's requirement for assistance relates to decision making, behavior control, and acquiring knowledge and skills. The communication relationship is still alternating between complementary and symmetrical patterns with the balance toward symmetrical relationships.

These systems are presented in the form of a model (Fig. 7–1) to highlight the fact that as clients move along the illness–wellness continuum, the nature of complementary–symmetrical communication patterns change.

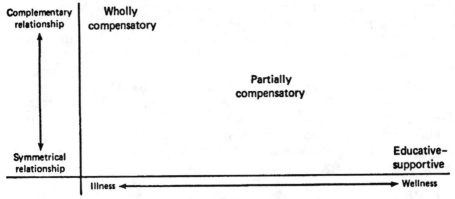

Figure 7–1. Orem's three nursing systems.

Illness–Wellness Continuum

As clients move along the continuum from illness to wellness they can move from a world of highly specialized technology with sophisticated monitoring and life-support systems to an environment of mutual decision making and control in which they regain their ability to assume self-care. The emphasis on life threatening physiological needs shifts to fulfillment of psychological or coping needs.

Psychological Aspects of Illness. There are characteristic psychological aspects that are often associated with illness states and transcend the specific illness symptomatology. They are summarized below:*

Illness	Wellness
Dependence	Independence
Passivity	Activeness
Heightened fear and anxiety	Lessened fear and anxiety
Self-rejection	Self-acceptance
Lowered feeling of self-worth	Strong feeling of self-worth
Identity loss and identity confusion	Sense of identity

In acute phases of illness, when clients are dependent and traditional health care (and cure) is given by others, there is heightened anxiety and concern. There is also a loss of roles and identity as a result both of removal from ordinary daily roles (worker, mother, father, friend, neighbor, child) and the anonymity of being a patient or client.

While a state of physical dependency is never a preferred state it is almost inevitable when a client is ill. The goal of the nurse–client relationship, however, is for the client to gain independence of functioning as rapidly as

*From Purtilo, 1984.

possible. The psychological aspects of illness are related to how illness is viewed in our culture, to the nature of the illness itself, to the role of being ill, or to some interaction of all three. They may be caused by the onset of the illness. The point here is that they lead to several kinds of client response that unless picked up by the nurse, can become barriers and inhibit effective and therapeutic communication.

Sociological Aspects of Illness. The "sick role" is taken on by clients who consider themselves ill under the following conditions: first, clients are incapacitated through no fault of their own; second, clients exhibit a desire to get well and to return to normal functioning within the limits of their capacities; and finally, clients express their desire to get well by cooperating with physicians and nurses (Enelow & Swisher, 1986).

Incapacities may also be viewed by clients and/or nurses as caused by the clients themselves through neglect or failure to take responsibility of their illness. In these cases, clients are not necessarily exempt from disapproval and in some instances can feel remorse and guilt.

Nurses and clients can have difficulty differentiating between taking responsibility for one's illness and assuming responsibility for one's health. They may believe that illness can be a punishment for sins and that somehow clients are to blame for what has occurred. Most of us have done this at some level in our lives, believing, for example, that we deserve the consequences of a sore throat and fever for not taking adequate care of ourselves and coming down with a cold.

Complementary–Symmetrical Relationship Continuum

Nurse–client dyads in wholly compensatory systems are complementary; the nurse assumes a superior role and the client an inferior role in the communication interaction. The psychological aspects associated with illness listed on pages 156–157 are characteristic of clients who are totally incapacitated physically and whose environment is controlled by nurses. Such comments as "It is time to turn on your other side" or "I am giving you a medication in your left buttock to help you breathe more easily" do not encourage active responses from clients.

The expression of client feelings and attitudes in wholly compensatory systems can present a challenge to nurses. Remember that feelings and attitudes are conveyed more strongly through nonverbal rather than verbal messages in dyadic communication. At the same time, one study (Preston, 1977) demonstrated that the major form of communication initiated by the nurse in wholly compensatory systems was "verbal questioning" and "giving directions." Responses by seriously ill clients were usually emblems such as head nods, hand movements, or facial expressions.

These responses may be the only ones clients are capable of making in a state of serious illness due to their physical condition. At the same time, they may represent a high degree of stress and fear on the part of clients. Nurses should pay attention to the "emblematic" responses of clients and be prepared to respond with empathy and care, not just with verbal directions. The client's inability to respond with words does not mean he or she is unfeeling or cannot benefit from care, concern, and other forms of therapeutic communication discussed in Chapter 4 of this book.

In addition, some unique complementary communication patterns between nurses and clients have been observed. Garvin (1981) identified 13 patterns of communication in complementary relationships in the hospital setting. In the following case situation, the 13 patterns are listed in the left-hand column with examples of each pattern demonstrated in the interactions in the right-hand column. As you read the following examples of interactions that demonstrate these 13 complementary patterns, think about the benefits and potential shortcomings of each.

Barbara Hall, a 37-year-old mother of three children, is a 1-day postoperative hysterectomy client for carcinoma-in-situ of the endometrium. The head nurse, during her morning rounds, is checking Barbara's dressing and fluid intake and output.

Complementary Pattern	Interaction
1. The nurse talks first.	*Nurse:* Barbara, I want to check your dressing.
2. The nurse selects the first topic in the first utterance.	*Client:* O.K.
3. The nurse asks questions: the client answers questions.	*Nurse:* How do you feel? Do you still have some pain? *Client:* No, not really.
4. When the nurse asks about a topic, the client is obliged to pursue the topic.	*Nurse:* Are you drinking plenty of water and fluids? *Client:* Well I had some orange juice with my breakfast a couple of minutes ago.
5. Topics in complementary interactions have to do with personal information regarding the client.	*Nurse:* Do you have any pain in your abdomen? (Puts hand on Mrs. Hall's lower abdomen to feel for urinary retention.)
6. When the client has answered the question, the nurse can then ask the same or similar question.	*Client:* Yes, a little. *Nurse:* Does this hurt? (Puts slight pressure on abdomen with hand.)
7. The nurse may ask a question and without waiting for a reply may ask a second question.	*Nurse:* Have you been sitting up on the edge of the bed? . . . Has your nurse told you that you have orders to sit up three times today?

Complementary Pattern	Interaction
	Client: I have trouble sitting up.
8. The nurse may verbally evaluate or revise the answer or response of the client in the next turn.	*Nurse:* You can sit up easily. You mean you have pain when you sit up.
	Client: I guess you are right.
9. The nurse proposes membership categories which is accepted by the client.	*Nurse:* Did you talk to Dr. Jackson? She is the chief surgical resident.
	Client: Is she the one that comes in to see me early in the morning?
10. The nurse manages the timing of the episode by using bracket markers. (Examples of bracket markers are "Now then," "Well," "O.K.")	*Nurse:* Yes. O.K. I'll check on you again before I go home.
11. The client uses a more formal term of address than the nurse.	*Client:* Nurse, you seem to know about . . .
12. The nurse may interrupt the client's talk before a transition relevant cue occurs.	*Nurse* (interrupting): Barbara, have you thought about going home?
	Client: No.
13. Nurse initiates closing of the episode.	*Nurse:* I'll see you later.

There are some points to be emphasized in the above interactions. The nurse (or person in superior role) controls the interaction time by starting, pacing and timing the interaction. Also, the nurse aggressed on the client's space by using her first name when the client did not call the nurse by her first name. The nurse controlled the content by selecting topics, asking questions, and choosing content of a personal nature. The nurse's expectations were that the client will answer questions relative to what is being asked.

In considering the benefits and potential problems in complementary communication, we want to stress again that the nature of the illness can play a role in complementary relationships, so it is difficult to evaluate these interactions on the same basis as those of two interactants who are healthy. As clients progress from illness to wellness states, they gain greater control and the relationship moves away from complementary toward symmetry. As was previously stated, complementary relationships are not necessarily negative; they help to provide one means for clients to get well. Thus, they serve a purpose. As students learn in teacher–student or children in parent–child complementary relationships, clients are assisted by the nurse to achieve wellness.

The important issue here is that nurses impart a concern of caring, empathy, and trust. If these complementary relationships become rigid and inflexible, the implication is that there will be more control over clients who want to please, to do the "right" thing. If the dyadic relationship is locked into one pattern, rather than alternating between complementary and symmetrical patterns, defensive behaviors can surface. For example, the nurse can blame, while the client placates. Healthy nurse–client dyads are dynamic and progress through phases (depending on the nature of the illness) in which both participants assume different roles. The goal of nursing care is to progress from doing everything *for* the client to assisting the client and finally, to planning *with* the client so that he or she can assume total responsibility for his or her health.

As the nurse–client dyad moves toward an equal or symmetrical pattern (or even a complementary relationship in which the client is one-up), greater demands are placed on nurses in terms of the complexity of the communication required.

Barriers to Effective Nurse–Client Communication

Nurses, as well as others, often use role labels to categorize clients. It is one way of *selectively* choosing what they want to perceive and represents an economy of effort in the complex process of perception. With the multitude of stimuli in health care settings that compete for nurses' attention, it is not difficult for them to fall into the habit of stereotyping. Placing persons into categories can help nurses to confront difficult situations more easily.

Unfortunately, stereotyping (or labeling, as it is commonly called) limits effective communication. Labels are based on erroneous (or at least inappropriate) concepts about persons and how they *ought* to behave. For example, nurses who assume either consciously or unconsciously that *all* older persons are disoriented will certainly be less effective in communicating with these clients than nurses who regard older individuals as "unique." In addition to the elderly, other types of clients who can easily fall prey to labeling are "the alcoholic," "the terminally ill," "the confused," "the incapacitated," and "the long-term chronic" client.

The "Hostile Client" Label. Persons who become ill respond in ways that can be a considerable burden to those around them. One of these responses is hostility, which is often directed at others. These clients have been characterized as "unhappy with their treatment," "unpleasant to talk to," "unappreciative," "manipulative," "uncooperative," "stubborn," as well as having a tendency of not following the hospital rules (Kelly & May, 1982; Alpert & Wittenberg, 1986). They refuse to accept the "illness role." They may also be destructive clients who communicate poorly. Their behavior in a hospital setting is characterized by constant demands such as using the call light, frequently asking for a bedpan, or complaining about the hospital food.

Hostile behavior can be difficult for the nurse to interpret accurately. Unfortunately, hostile behavior can lead to stereotyping these clients as "demanding," "malingering," "complaining," or "bad patient." These descriptions are a form of blaming the client. The labeling of clients in this manner can also become a self-fulfilling prophecy: that is, nurses will reinforce the behavior of such clients by responding only to complaints or demands, which will then lead to further demands and complaints.

Once a client receives a negative label, the label can permeate the entire nursing staff of a unit, making it all the more difficult for the client to change. Many nurses remember the classic film *Mrs. Reynolds Needs a Nurse*. The film depicts an elderly woman who is acutely ill and has become a major problem on the unit, with her constant demands, numerous complaints, and overall hostile attitude towards nurses, doctors, and other health workers. The situation gradually worsens until a student nurse arrives on the scene. She actively "listens" to Mrs. Reynolds and begins to understand the reasons underlying her negative behavior. The film is a particularly moving one, as it hits at the heart of nursing. Although there was therapeutic nurse–client communication, the student had to *change the attitude* of an entire staff on the unit toward Mrs. Reynolds in order to change the client's behavior.

In terms of handling hostile clients, the nurse first needs to be accepting of the client. Nurses who know and understand themselves *as well as* the clients they are working with are able to accept such idiosyncratic behaviors and traits. It is important for nurses to be aware of their own personal biases as well as cultural and gender differences in their clients (Alpert & Wittenberg, 1986). Using communication skills of understanding, empathy, and support, they can begin to understand and, in turn, help clients to alter their behavior.

The "Good Patient" Label. A more difficult problem to detect is the client who has, at some level, decided *not* to be a burden on the staff and suffers in silence. These clients have been described as "amusing," "optimistic," "cheerful," and "grateful" (Kelly & May, 1982). They abide by the rules and do not question or assert. They joke and laugh with the nurses. They mutually cooperate with nurses to set goals aimed toward wellness. Good clients are often highly motivated to recover from illness.

In terms of Satir's communication styles, these clients may placate by assuring the nurse they feel fine when, in actuality, they have pain. There may be a contradiction between verbal and body language messages, although an accomplished "good patient" can be quite successful in disguising inner feelings from the message that is communicated to the nurse.

The major difficulty with the "good patients" involves detecting them. The "good patient" may go unnoticed because it requires direct intervention to uncover the client's problems. The cues that indicate the client is suffering, such as a slight grimace or hesitation in answering a question, may be subtle. Also, nurses who are feeling harried may only apply oil to "the wheel that squeaks the loudest"; this will never be the "good patient."

The "good patient" is rewarded for "good patient" behavior by smiles, compliments, and overheard messages. For example, a client may overhear, "That's Mrs. Williams, she is always smiling, even though she just had surgery." For all of these reasons, the "good patient" is difficult to uncover.

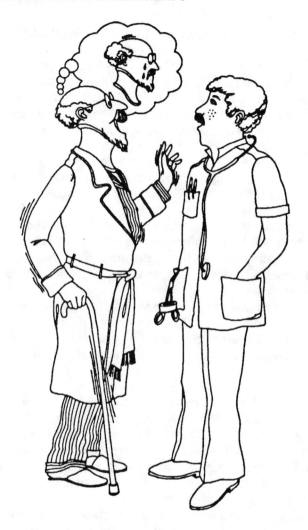

The following exercise is designed to help you learn how to discover the "good patient."

THE "GOOD PATIENT" EXERCISE

1. Pair up. One partner will be A, the other B.
2. A pretends to be a client recovering at home from an illness (stroke or a heart attack). B will be checking up on A's recovery. A will act as if everything is all right, but in one aspect pretend to be the "good patient." That is, A will "cover up" some problem, but will give subtle

clues that things are not all right.
3. *B* interviews *A* as if doing a checkup.
4. *B* listens to *A*, watching for the following nonverbal cues:
    a. Eye contact
    b. Facial expression
    c. Body movements (posture)
    d. Tone of voice
5. *A* and *B* switch roles.
6. Share experiences with each other. Were either of you able to figure out when the other was being the "good patient?" If so, what were the cues?

The "Good Nurse" Label

The "good nurse" tends to be task-oriented rather than person-oriented. This nurse can give top priority to high-visibility tasks, at times, to the detriment of client care, as shown in the following story.

> A nursing instructor we know was hospitalized for a thyroidectomy. She was told that she had a p.r.n. postop pain medication ordered. The first evening after the operation she was experiencing considerable pain. She saw the medication nurse passing out medications in the room across the hallway and asked if she might have her p.r.n. medication as she was in some pain. The nurse said that she had to finish one side of the hallway and then work up the other side and after that, then she would bring her the medication, a task that might take anywhere from 30 minutes to more than an hour.

This situation, as ridiculous as it sounds, is not uncommon. The nurse was totally consumed with carrying out the task to the exclusion of caring for the client.

The "good nurse" is always busy, always carrying out the doctors' orders and usually feels overworked. The "good nurse" rarely stops to listen, *really* listen to clients. There is a tendency to be superreasonable or a bit blaming. The overall orientation of the "good nurse" to nursing is similar to a computerized exercise in which the nurse collects, analyzes, and produces data. The "humanistic" approach to the client is nonexistent. "Good nurses" hide behind the armor of a stereotype not only to avoid their own self-disclosure, but to prevent clients from sharing their feelings and experiences in stressful situations.

Clients, on the other hand, consistently emphasize the caring aspect of nurses (rather than their technical ability) when recalling good care in stressful illness experiences. The consumer's concern about nurses' credentials is less likely to be of concern than adequacy of health care received. Client's perception of the nursing role is still primarily focused on personal qualities rather than technical abilities or skills (Brooks & Kleine-Kracht, 1983). As a medical school professor who had a laryngectomy recently stated to one of the authors, "The most important thing was that the nurse cared" (Newman, 1985).

Unfortunately, "good patients" reinforce "good nurses." Clients who do not wish to "take up a nurse's time," "cause trouble," "call a nurse if they can do something by themselves," (in spite of doctor's orders), or look on the nurse as busy and overworked (oftentimes true) help to foster the stereotyped role of the "good nurse."

Fortunately, recent research indicates that time spent with clients is not related to whether the client is "good" or "bad" in the eyes of the nurses. Also there is some question as to whether nurses (and physicians) actually label clients by their good and bad qualities. The above stereotypes have been presented to use as warning indicators; that is, when other nurses (as well as yourself) are using these labels, something is not right.

The reality is that there are no "easy" clients. Fear, pain, and discouragement can be present even in a simple diagnosis. The interactive nature of the nurse–client relationship should impede the use of labeling. Clients who can assume an *active* role as a *participant* in the decision-making process related to health goals are not usually labeled good, bad, or anything else.

Working on Mutuality: Problem Solving and Contracting

We have previously discussed the need for mutuality in the nurse's work with clients. This includes the need for both parties to work on achievement of goals as well as goal setting. This can be accomplished through the use of problem solving or contracting.

Problem solving is a task that confronts every person in daily life situations. From the moment we wake up in the morning, we are confronted with many decisions, however, we usually do not go through a series of steps to arrive at these decisions. In nurse–client encounters, problem solving is deliberate and objective. Clients need help in setting realistic and appropriate goals to bring about change. A problem-solving model is systematic and can be used to help the client solve his or her own problems.

Problem–Solving Model

- The problem is presented.
- The problem is defined and/or refined.
- Define specific criteria that ascertain if the problem is solved.
- Solutions and/or options are listed.
- Solutions and/or options are prioritized and/or decided.
- One option is tried.

- The option is evaluated (did it work?).
- Recycle if necessary.

The model presented is a step-by-step process of inquiry which helps to facilitate the solution of the problem. The problem-solving methodology and nursing process are very similar in that each presents a systematic step-by-step methodology for arriving at the solution of the problem; the problem is presented (assessment), the solutions are prioritized (plan), one option is tried (implementation), and the solution is evaluated (evaluation). The problem-solving method presents a planned approach to help clients ventilate problems, and the orientation is client-centered.

When they begin to use a problem-solving model, nurses often say, "I just can't get clients to say what is really bothering them." Problem definition is often the most difficult step in the problem-solving process. Once the problem is properly defined, which may require extensive discussion and examination of related issues, the subsequent phases of the problem-solving model are more easily handled. When nurses begin to use the problem-solving model, they often find that the most difficult step is refining and defining the problem. Once the problem is defined, which may require extensive discussion and examination of related issues, the subsequent phases of the problem-solving model are more easily handled.

The Use of Client Contracting

One of the ways nurses are beginning to help clients participate in their own health is to use client contracting, in which clients actually write down the specific steps or activities they will complete as part of their health care. The processes involved in devising a behavioral contract can be quite complex and are beyond the scope of this book. The central idea of contracting, however, includes appreciating the principle of reinforcement, that is, that behavior is controlled by its consequences (Steckel, 1980). Nurses wishing for a client to increase a form of self-care need to build in sensible and desirable rewards (positive consequences) for activities that promote health of the client.

Nurses are frequently presented with fairly complicated sets of behavior for the client to manage, such as the changes in functioning for the client who has had a stroke and is planning to go home. One way of identifying complex behavior changes which have been linked to a nursing goal is to break each behavior down into small systematic steps. These steps leading to desired behavior must be observable and measurable. Also, specific rewards, for example, treating oneself to a new article of clothing, a meal out, or a minivacation, should be built into the contract as a reward for completing various parts of the needed procedures. By working with the client to develop a meaningful and useful contract, the nurse can help the client identify his or her own priorities for health care and increase the probability of success for a given regimen.

CONCLUSION

The nurse's role has evolved over the past 150 years from "helping the patient suffering from disease" in Nightingale's era to the diagnosis and treatment of human responses in the 1980s. Today, the nurse's role is typified as a collaborative one. It includes specialized functions and activities related to wellness as well as illness. Concepts such as health education, prevention, compliance, and health promotion are important parts of today's nurse's thinking and activities.

Many forces and influences in the health care system have created greater demands on the ability of nurses to communicate effectively with clients. The nurse's role has changed from the traditional bedside nurturing and caring of physically and psychologically dependent clients to that of mutual relationships. The client's role changed in a series of phases, from a passive to an active one in which he or she assumes the responsibility for the setting of goals by utilizing a problem-solving methodology.

Enlisting client participation and addressing health issues that promote wellness are central goals to the professional framework of nursing practice. Nurses who pay particular attention to the quality of interaction with clients will find themselves less likely to use ineffective labels or stereotypes of clients.

The use of problem solving and behavioral contracting are two ways to increase effective communication between nurse and client.

REFERENCES

Alpert, J. S., & Wittenberg, S. M. *A clinician's companion.* Boston: Little, Brown, & Co., 1986.

Armstrong, D. The fabrication of nurse-patient relationships. *Social Science & Medicine,* 1983, 17(8), 457–460.

Artinian, B. M. Implementation of the intersystem patient–care model in clinical practice. *Journal of Advanced Nursing,* 1983, 8, 117–124.

Brooks, J. A., & Kleine-Kracht, A. E. Evolution of a definition of nursing. *Advances in Nursing Science,* 1983, 5(4), 51–85.

Caporael-Katz, B. Health, self-care and power: Shifting the balance. *Topics in Clinical Nursing,* October 1983.

Enelow, A. J., & Swisher, S. N. *Interviewing and patient care* (3rd ed.). New York: Oxford University Press, 1986.

Garvin, B. Rules for creating health care relationships through talk. ERIC document 206019, May 1981.

Kasch, C. Interpersonal competence and communication in the delivery of nursing care. *Advances in Nursing Science,* 1984, 6(2), 71–88.

Kelly, M. P., & May, D. Good and bad patients: A review of the literature and a theoretical critique. *Journal of Advanced Nursing*, 1982, 7, 147–156.

King, I. *A theory for nursing.* New York: Wiley, 1981.

Newman, J. Personal interview. January 17, 1985.

Orem, D. *Nursing: Concepts of practice* (3rd ed.). New York: McGraw-Hill, 1985.

Preston, A. *Communication dynamics of ventilator dependent patients.* Master's Thesis (unpublished), University of Illinois, 1977.

Steckel, S. B. Contracting with patient-selected reinforcers. *American Journal of Nursing.* 1980, 80(9), 1596–1599.

8 Nurse–Coworker Dyads

BEHAVIORAL OBJECTIVES

By reading this chapter and participating in the exercises, students will be able to:

1. Identify four dimensions of reciprocal nurse–coworker relationships
2. Demonstrate an understanding of three major factors that create barriers to effective communication in nurse–aide relationships
3. Analyze the key aspects of the nurse–physician relationship that affect communication
4. Relate issues of territoriality with nurse–physician collaboration
5. Discuss how the formation of co-territory enhances collaboration between nurses and physicians

The nurse rarely exists as a totally independent health care provider. Today's nurse interacts professionally as well as personally with a wide range of coworkers, including aides, clerks, pharmacists, physicians, psychologists, medical technicians, social workers, and health educators, as well as with other nurses.

This chapter includes the major coworker relationships encountered in health settings (nurse–aide and nurse–physician), and raises some general issues pertaining to communication between nurses and other coworkers. Effective strategies with coworkers, as well as physicians, are also discussed.

Four Dimensions of Reciprocal Nurse–Coworker Relationships

Even with improved role relationships, if communication relationships between nurses and other coworkers are to be effective, they must be "reciprocal," that is, mutual or shared interactions (Phillips, 1979). Such interactions imply openness, equality, and the opportunity to present one's information or point of view without being blamed. The state of reciprocity can be measured across four dimensions: task, authority, deference, and affect. These four dimensions, which provide a framework for examining nurse–coworker relationships, were first conceptualized by Stevenson (1977) and adapted to nurse–physician relationships by Phillips (1979).

Task Dimension. The task dimension relates to the division of tasks or activities delegated to the particular health care provider; what client care tasks should be relegated to the nurse, the physician, or the social worker? History shows that many tasks have shifted among these professionals. For example, physical assessment of the heart, a task that was once exclusively carried out by the physician is now within the realm of the nurse.

Authority Dimension. The authority dimension relates to how much power each health care provider has in relation to other health professionals, that is, which health care provider is at the top of the "pecking order" in the eyes of the other health care provider groups. The amount of power one has is usually determined by the amount of education or knowledge one possesses.

Deference Dimension. The deference dimension is related to whose needs take precedence, the client's or the health care provider's. It is important that there be a reciprocal relationship between the health care providers if the client's needs are to be met. If everyone's opinions on what is best for the client are heard, then the decisions made are based on shared decisions. In this way a "therapeutic community" is created and the client benefits, especially if the client requires long-term care.

Affect Dimension. The affect dimension is concerned with the feelings that health care providers have toward each other. Health providers are able to coordinate their efforts more effectively for the ultimate benefit of the client when they work in an environment of mutual respect for each other's role or profession.

Reciprocal relationships between the nurse and other health care providers begin with a respect for oneself. One needs a sense of self-worth not only to be emotionally supportive of clients, but to be able to work within health care environments with others.

THE NURSE–AIDE ROLE RELATIONSHIP

The nurse–aide relationship is rarely addressed in the nursing literature. Aides usually have a clearcut definition of tasks or activities. They are often experienced in these tasks, having worked in a particular health care setting longer than the nurse. Normally, aides do not question the nurse's authority; they know they are at the bottom of the "pecking order."

Three major factors that create barriers to effective communication between the nurse (team leader or head nurse) and the aide; first, the aide does not always know what the nurse expects; second, the aide may feel that no credit is given for good judgment; and third, the aide may feel that nurse coworkers avoid giving help to aides.

In the first barrier, expectations in terms of tasks, the aide is stating that there is little opportunity to clarify expectations; that there is no reciprocity in the relationship. While the aide can be a constant in a health care setting, the leaders can change. Each nursing leader has different priorities. Thus, the aide plays a "guessing game" as to what the particular nurse in charge expects of him or her. In nurse–aide interaction, the "what," "when," and "how" are sometimes given, but the "why" omitted. The following two statements by the nurse to the aide demonstrate the difference between omitting and including the "why."

Mrs. O'Brien, the aide, has the task of filling the water pitchers on the unit. The nurse in charge might say to her:

Statement A: Do *not* fill the water pitcher of the client in Room 202.
Statement B: Do not give Mr. O'Hara, the client in Room 202, any liquids. He is on n.p.o. because he is on call for surgery.

In statement *A*, the nurse did not give a "why"; the aide concluded there must be a reason that the nurse did not want to tell her, and she attempted to fill in the answer herself (by thinking the nurse was angry with Mr. O'Hara). In statement *B*, the aide was given an explanation which would help her perform a simple task dependably because of the rationale given for the action.

The second barrier, the lack of credit for the aide's good judgment, demonstrates an absence of reciprocity in the nurse–aide relationship, particularly in the affect dimension. While the aide is expected to accept and respect the nurse, there is little sense of being respected in turn by the nurse. A word of thanks or praise by the nurse about the aide's performance is essential.

The third barrier, no help from the nurse, demonstrates a lack of reciprocity across the deference dimension. The aide thinks that the nurse who does not help is placing a greater priority on serving a superior such as the head nurse or physician. The following is a common occurrence in the hospital setting:

The aide is carrying out a procedure for a client (taking a temperature and pulse) and the call light flashes in the next room. The aide notes that the nurse at the nurses' station does not answer the light. When the aide answers the light, the aide sees the nurse sitting at the nurses' station desk charting. The aide assumes that the nurse *does not want* to answer the light, that his or her role in the eyes of the nurse is not important, and that he or she is not being recognized. Satisfaction with the role of the aide begins to diminish.

The aide often receives an assignment on a written assignment sheet, but other than that, all directives are verbal and often one way. There is no provision for aides to respond even if they do not understand the orders. Effective nurse leaders take the time and opportunity to communicate face-to-face with aides, utilizing all channels. They also include aides in the planning of client care. A perceptive aide who has had contact with the client for long periods of time will often be able to come up with solutions to client care problems that are creative and useful. In addition, if aides are included in the planning of care, they will feel that what they are doing is important and that they themselves are appreciated.

THE NURSE–HEALTH PROFESSIONAL ROLE RELATIONSHIP

The major purpose of nurse–coworker communication is to share and exchange information about the client and to make joint decisions. Nurse–coworker communication relationships are, theoretically, symmetrical. There is reciprocity in the relationship, with mutual agreement on a goal, that goal being to enable the client to function independently. The task dimension of each health care provider often overlaps with a nursing task; for example, the social worker and the nurse both interview the client and often seek the same information from the client. Often coworkers and nurses are not aware of expertise overlap or how much difference in perspective each has in his or her approach to client care.

In the ideal nurse–coworker relationship, each partner excels in a particular area of expertise and works collaboratively in exercising the expertise to the benefit of the client. They both work to serve client needs (deference dimension); they also respect each other's opinion, as well as have mutual respect for the particular profession that the other represents (affect dimension).

EXERCISE IN COMMUNICATION WITH OTHER HEALTH PROFESSIONALS

For each of the following situations, think about how you could use each of the communication skills listed below it to insure the quality of client care, efficient information exchange, and heightened self-worth of both the nurse and the other. Use either Chapters 4 and 5 to refresh your memory of the skills if necessary. Some suggested uses of the skills are found on the right side of the page. Cover them until you have answered and then compare them. Even as there are several skills that can be brought to each situation, there are many ways to use each skill.

SITUATION 1
An aide comes up to you while you are busy with a client and asks you a question that could wait: "What time is Mr. Brown supposed to be ambulated?"

Skill	Suggested Option
Clarification	Is something wrong with him now?
"I" message	I'm busy right now and will get to you when I can. (Said *without* blame.)
Reflection	You seem concerned about Mr. Brown.
Verbal/nonverbal reassurance	(Touch shoulder) Thank you for reminding me. I'll get to it in a minute.

SITUATION 2

A physician comes over to you and asks a question about a new client you know little about. How do you handle it?

Skill	Suggested Option
"I" statement	I'm a little short on information. The client is new.
Paraphrase	You want to know _____. (Paraphrase the question.) I'll have to find out.

SITUATION 3

The social worker comes over to you and starts discussing a client with a complicated illness. It becomes obvious that the social worker does not have full information or understanding about the illness; she then asks: "Well, what is the prognosis—what should I tell the family?" How would you handle this?

Skill	Suggested Option
Focused question	How much do you know about the illness?
"I" message	I feel we ought to talk about the illness first.
"Why" question (not recommended)	Why do you want to know that?

Each of these recommended skills represents a beginning to what could be useful communication. Can you also see what the negative consequences of blaming, placating, "why" questions, or patronizing might be?

THE NURSE–PHYSICIAN ROLE RELATIONSHIP

The nurse–physician relationship is one of the most challenging role issues in nursing. The focus of each profession, the changing roles of the nurse, and issues related to territory previously discussed in this book all interact to create opportunities for conflict as well as cooperation and collaboration.

The primary concern of both nursing and medicine is the client's health–illness state. How each profession carries out its respective role has differed over the last several decades. While there has always been a degree of overlap in functions between the two professions, the focus of each has been unique. In recent years, this overlap has been more pronounced, with nursing assuming many of the functions that were originally the strict domain of medicine.

Four elements of a positive relationship between nurses and physicians are: mutual trust and respect, open communication, a willingness to cooperate with each other, and competence in performance of one's role. In one study, the majority of 1044 nurses and 536 physicians from 15 different hospitals nationwide perceived the nurse–physician relationship in the hospital setting as "positive" (69% of nurses and 70% of physicians); 15% of the nurses and 14% of the physicians described the relationship as "mixed," and 8% of the nurses and 2% of physicians felt the relationship was "mostly poor" (Prescott & Bowen, 1985).

An additional finding from this study was that disagreement between nurses and physicians is not necessarily perceived as negative. Indeed, it can be a necessary and healthy aspect of nurse–physician communication. Nurses and physicians have differing perspectives on many client-care problems and these perspectives are based on different but complementary orientations of the two disciplines as well as the different types of information to which each profession is exposed. If both professions continue to adopt attitudes of mutual respect for each other, more collaboration will occur. From our experience, physicians find it most difficult to *listen* to nurses, while nurses find it most difficult to *talk* to physicians. An example follows:

Leslie Shaw, a staff nurse in a neurosurgical unit, was informed by her nurse manager that Dr. English, one of the neurosurgeons, wanted to see her. Leslie's reaction was one of anxiety: "What have I done wrong?" she asked herself. The next day, when she saw Dr. English on the unit, he stated to her that he had met a family relative in another city and was bringing her greetings!

Self-worth, which was threatened in Leslie's case, is essential in order to communicate effectively with physicians. Self-worth can be affected differently by various role relationships. For example, a nurse may feel very good about clinical skills and nurse–client interactions and have a low self-image or feel threatened when presenting information to physicians or even when giving instructions to aides. The following exercise is designed to help you begin to raise your self-worth as a nurse.

EXERCISE IN INCREASING YOUR SELF-WORTH

1. Break up into groups of four.
2. Think of three traits, talents, or actions that you feel are positive or good about yourself in relation to your nursing role; for example, "I am well organized in my client care," "the other nurses like me because I am always willing to help out."
3. Write your three positive items on paper.
4. Share with the group.
5. Review and discuss. How difficult was this exercise? If it was difficult, was your own *low* self-worth getting in the way?

Now that you have listed your strengths, do you feel more positive about yourself?

Two factors that have had an impact on the nurse–physician role relationship are salaries and setting.

Salaries. Since 1945, the gap between physicians' and nurses' salaries has increased dramatically. After World War II, nurses' salaries were approximately one-third those of physicians; today they are less than one-fifth those of physicians (Mechanic & Aiken, 1982). Obviously, this does not foster a collegial relationship between nurses and physicians. The recent trend for increased salaries for nurses is a welcome sign.

Setting. One characteristic of professionals is that they have a strong sense of calling or motivation to their chosen profession. It can be difficult for nurses to feel this sense of calling, particularly in the acute care setting where over 60 percent of all nurses work. How does one feel a sense of calling if the setting in which one is employed requires night and weekend work hours, high levels of stress associated with the job, and at the same time one's contribution to the job is undervalued by one's coworkers in the health care setting?

Nurse–Physician Collaboration

Nurses and physicians will have role-related problems as long as clients exist. Many of these problems relate to professional overlap, for example, terms such as "joint practice" or "nursing diagnosis" can be threatening to physicians who do not understand the full intent of their meaning. The use of such charged words without taking time to communicate their meaning can create conflict.

The concepts presented in Chapter 6 on territoriality can provide insight into the issues underlying nurse–physician conflict and collaboration. Consider the following example:

A client is in acute distress and needs a blood replacement. The nurse is required to stay with the client. A physician comes by and orders the blood. He then asks the nurse to go to the blood bank to pick it up. The nurse tells the physician that she is required to stay with the client and cannot leave the unit to get the blood.

What kind of response did the nurse use in the above situation? Before one can answer that question, several issues related to territory should be examined.

One dimension of territoriality is *action territory* or the sense of ownership related to a sphere of authority, expertise, or activity. This is territory which includes all functions related to one's work role (Shaw, 1983). As employees of a hospital, there are certain privileges, rights, and responsibilities that are inherent in the nurse's and physician's roles. In the above example, the nurse is performing an expected role when the physician asks a favor. Thus, the physician has *aggressed* on the nurse's territory, an action that is within his rights.

In the above example, the nurse asserted and defended her action territory by telling the physician she could not leave the unit. The nurse defended the action territory including the rights and privileges that go along with the role.

Why would any nurse respond to the physician's request that is clearly beyond the limits of his or her role? The nurse's job description does not include trips to the blood bank to pick up blood; indeed an implicit role function of the nurse is to remain within close call of critically ill clients. To leave the unit would be inappropriate behavior.

There are, however, several reasons why some nurses might be tempted to act inappropriately in this situation. One is simply "liking" to do others favors. Another reason why a nurse might be tempted to do what the physician requested is that she or he wants something in exchange. Perhaps the nurse in the example is thinking that at a later time, the physician will do something in return for the favor. A third reason is that some nurses feel threatened by physicians and placate as an attempt to handle the stress that unreasonable requests create.

EXERCISE IN TERRITORIALITY AND NURSE–PHYSICIAN INTERACTIONS

Pair up and look at the following situations which occur in the clinical setting. As you read each situation, define the nurse's action territory. Then look at the nurse's response. Was it an assertive or aggressive response? How does the response fit into the ideas of territory presented in this book? Discuss what you might do in similar circumstances with your partner. Attempt to uncover your own preferences in communication (asserting, being aggressive, even being passive) as well as thinking about the implications of your responses to these and other difficult situations you may encounter in your nursing experience.

Situation	Response
A physician interrupts your work and asks, "Where is Mrs. Jones' chart?"	You stop what you are doing and look for it.
A physician examining a chart complains in an abusive manner that the results of the x-rays he ordered 3 days ago are not on the chart.	You take the physician aside and state that you do not wish to be spoken to in such a manner.
You are performing a sterile procedure and need one more package of sterile dressings opened. A physician walks in the room.	You prefer to wait, rather than ask the physician to open the package.
The client's pain medication does not appear to be effective following his or her surgery.	You call the physician and request a change in the pain medication for the client.
A physician has written an order that arouses your curiosity of why it is being given.	You question the physician about the order.
A physician calls over the telephone from surgery for you to inform a client's family that the preliminary pathological report of the biopsy is positive.	You tell the physician that you wish him or her to inform the client of the biopsy report.

Nurse–physician interactions, such as those in the examples above, can lead to conflict when disagreement exists on the nature of the role relationship between the two participants. An example is when the nurse perceives him- or herself as a peer or equal while at the same time the physician perceives him- or herself in a superior position. If the interaction is a symmetrical one in which both parties not only understand the role, but mutually agree to the role boundaries, then there is no conflict. If one party, however, considers him- or herself in a complementary role, that is, a superior position, and the other does not agree to this complementary role, then conflict arises.

There have been significant changes in the nurse–physician relationship. In the past, the traditional role relationship between nurses and physicians was a complementary one, characterized by dominance–submission. This relationship was often portrayed as a power struggle, especially in the arena of clinical decision-making. While these stereotypic relationships between physician and nurse still exist in some situations, their incidence and importance have been exaggerated by the television media. In general, physician–nurse interactions occur at a high professional level (Alpert & Wittenberg, 1986).

The ambiguity that exists today in the nurse–physician role relationship is often related to rules which govern the relationship. Many nurses are stating convincingly that they are colleagues in a *symmetrical* relationship. This is especially true with nurse practitioners or nurse clinicians, where nurses have specialized competence. At the same time, there can be obvious differences in skill, educational status, income, and responsibility between, for example, the head of surgery at a hospital and a newly graduated baccalaureate nurse. This raises one of the most fascinating role relation issues for health providers, namely, how can collegiality be achieved between medicine and nursing?

Conditions for Collegiality. Nurses and physicians work best as colleagues when there is

- A willingness to adopt an *attitude* of mutual respect
- Mutual trust for each other's competence
- Cooperation and communication
- Support from the "system"

The goal of quality health care for the client is at the heart of both the nursing and medical professions. But what of the status of equality in personal interactions? While nurses perceive the nurse–physician dyad as an alternating symmetrical–complementary relationship, some physicians still view the relationship as totally complementary with no feedback for correction or control. This has resulted in conflicting views of the two roles.

There are instances in which nurses as a professional group have a poor self-image and do not have reciprocal relationships with physicians, especially in the dimensions of deference and affect. Many nurses perceive the physician–nurse relationship as a totally "one-up" relationship in which the physician makes the decisions.

The purpose of this section is *not* to state how things should be but to alert nurses to the fact that the doctor–nurse relationship is changing and varies considerably from setting to setting. When the nurse desires a high degree of independence or collegiality, communication problems may arise from differences of opinion between the physician and the nurse, implied superior relationship (or double messages) from the physician, or from incongruent and mixed messages from the nurse.

Co-Territoriality. One way to enable nurses to approach the contemporary issues of complementary–symmetrical role relationships and enhance nurse–

physician communication is to collaborate by *sharing* the territory or establishing a co-territory (Bigbee, 1984). The establishment of a co-territory ideally leads to increased security because neither nurse nor physician stands alone; rather, they form an alliance to share the territory and increase the size of their territory and simplify the management through a cooperative venture.

There are advantages of co-territory. The first is that the size of the territory through joint management is increased. The nurse and physician together can claim ownership to a larger action territory. The maintenance of the territory is facilitated through this joint management.

The establishment of a co-territory takes effort and time; time to negotiate and communicate with the persons who are sharing the territory. In co-territories persons also feel that they need approval for certain actions from the other persons within a given territory.

Bakker-Rabdau (1982) has suggested some basic rules for co-territory:

- You must do your work; if not then someone else has to do it for you.
- You must do your work according to the standards set by the group.
- You may not do someone else's work for him or her (unless they agree).
- If you do take over someone's work with their permission, then you have to do the job according to the level of competency set by him or her.

The concept of co-territory is closely related to collaboration, which is often embodied in a team approach to care. Collaboration encompasses an attitude of mutual respect and agreement in the task roles, competent performance, and cooperation and communication.

The response to the client to collaborative practice is overwhelmingly positive. Clients expect it today and assume it is occurring. The team approach to client health problems reduces unnecessary repetition, allowing for nursing and medicine roles to enhance each other. We believe co-territory is the most effective way for nurses to achieve greater control and autonomy in their practice as well as in the nursing profession as a whole.

The Nurse–Medical Student Role Relationship

Relating to the nurse–physician role is the nurse–medical student role. For the most part, nurses and medical students have limited interaction. The highest degree is usually before teaching rounds in the early A.M. which coincides with the morning report. The nurse and medical student, both preoccupied with respective tasks, do not really listen to one another nor share each other's concerns regarding patients. One study (Webster, 1985) highlighted the confusion that medical students have about nurses' roles in the hospital setting. As the students progressed through medical school, they were able to describe the role of the physician in more specific, clearer terms. Conversely, the role of the nurse became more diffuse! Again the lack of information about what nurses do influenced medical students' perception of the role of the nurse.

Emergence of the Nurse Practitioner

A new facet in the nurse–physician relationship is the emergence of the nurse practitioner. A nurse practitioner is a licensed registered nurse who has taken specialized training in primary care. Nurse practitioner programs leading to a degree are graduate-level programs. They give the nurse experience in physical assessment, treatment, and related health aspects of a specific client group such as children, families, or the elderly. The emergence of this type of graduate-level education carries with it the impetus for nurses to expect more equality in their dealings with physicians.

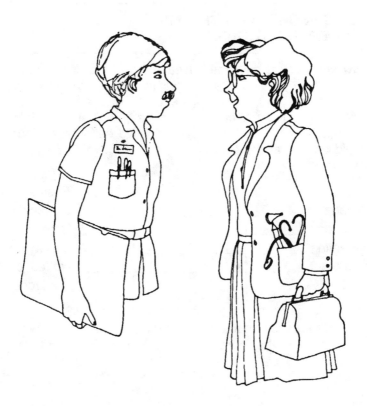

The question arises as to the differences in roles between nurse practitioners and physicians. The nurse practitioner is oriented towards a "caring" role and the physician is oriented towards a "curing" role. The caring role emphasizes behaviors such as emotional support, teaching, and listening, whereas the curing role focuses on the physical or treatment needs of the patient. Physicians can emphasize "care" and nurses can emphasize "cure"; however nursing studies have demonstrated that the caring orientation is central to most nursing interventions, (Brenner and Wrubel, 1989), and that patients look primarily to physicians regarding physical aspects of the illnesses (Beisecker et al., 1988).

While the focus of this chapter is on interactions between nurses and physicians, it is valuable to make frequent assessments of our own self-worth as we interact with others. By recognizing that our own self-worth is lowered in certain situations we can change our own behavior; this can result in doing things or communicating in such a way as to raise our level of self-worth and thus influence a solution to the problem.

The following exercise is designed to help you understand your feelings when relating to other professions.

EXERCISE IN SELF-WORTH AND COWORKER RELATIONSHIPS

1. How would you rate yourself on each of the following dimensions in terms of how you feel *when relating to a physician?* You can make an x in pencil on the appropriate line. (For example, if you felt a slight positive image, your mark might appear just to the right of the midline, but if you felt a strong negative self-image, your mark would appear at the extreme left near the words *Negative self-image*).

Negative self-image				Positive self-image
Unimportant				Important
Undeserving				Deserving
Fear of other				No fear of other
Judged by other				Not judged by other

2. Now rate yourself on the following dimensions as to how you feel about yourself when communicating with an aide or orderly.

Negative self-image				Positive self-image
Unimportant				Important
Undeserving				Deserving
Fear of other				No fear of other
Judged by other				Not judged by other

3. Now, rate yourself on the following dimensions as to how you feel about yourself when communicating with people from other health professions (social worker, psychologist, etc.)

Negative self-image				Positive self-image
Unimportant				Important
Undeserving				Deserving
Fear of other				No fear of other
Judged by other				Not judged by other

4. Compare your ratings in the three groupings. Which are different? Which are the same? What do you think made you rate yourself the way you did? If your responses were on the left side of the scales, what communication styles do you think you might use when you feel this way?

5. In the large group, discuss your answers to step 4 and answer the following questions:
   a. Is it necessary to feel superior or inferior in a hierarchical relationship?
   b. How is communication different when talking to a superior from talking to a subordinate?

CONCLUSION

Many issues influence communication between nurses and coworkers, including status, education, sex, race, and organizational concerns. One way of looking at many of these interactions is to consider their implications for territoriality. In addition, it may be prudent for nurses to be congruent and use their knowledge of communication channels and other skills in this book in attempting to handle difficult situations with coworkers. Finally, nurses should appreciate the needs for sharing responsibility for client care, be it in joint practice, shared leadership, or team delivery of health care. Even as nursing is becoming increasingly professional, it can, as a profession, be secure enough to work collaboratively with others in the health care system.

REFERENCES

Alpert, J. S., & Wittenberg, S. M. *A clinician's companion*. Boston: Little, Brown & Co., 1986.

Bakker-Rabdau, M. Workshop on assertion-aggression-affiliation. *Adult Development Program*, Peoria, Illinois, May, 1982.

Beisecker, A. E., Cobb, A. K., & Zeigler, D. K. *Archives of Neurology*. 1988, 45(5), 553–556.

Brenner, P. E., & Wrubel, J. *The primacy of caring*. Menlo Park, Calif.: Addison-Wesley Publishing, 1989.

Bigbee, J. Territoriality and prescriptive authority for nurse practitioners. *Nursing and Health Care*, 1984, 5(2), 106–110.

Mechanic, D., & Aiken, L. A cooperative agenda for medicine and nursing. *New England Journal of Medicine*, 1982, 307(12), 747–750.

Phillips, J. R. Health care provider relationships: A matter of reciprocity. *Nursing Outlook*, 1979, 27, 738–741.

Prescott, P. A., & Bowen, S. A. Physician–nurse relationships, *Annals of Internal Medicine*, 1985, 103, 127–133.

Shaw, R. *Privacy and action territory in a nursing home population*. M. S. Thesis (unpublished). University of Illinois, 1983.

Stevenson, J. S. *Issues and crises during middlescence*. New York: Appleton-Century-Crofts, 1977.

Webster, D. Medical students' views of the role of the nurse. *Nursing Research*, 1985, 34(5), 313–317.

Section III	# Communication and the Practice Setting

The third section of this book addresses communication between nurses and other members of the health care system within the context of the practice setting as well as with families and groups.

Nursing has traditionally been practiced in two settings: the hospital and the ambulatory care setting. With the advent of medical and nursing technology, hospitals and community outpatient agencies have been further subdivided into specialized categories. For example, in the hospital setting, there may be units for clients with acute illness (intensive care, coronary care, and renal dialysis units). Also, in spite of the fact that some ambulatory care units are located in the hospital, the client in such a unit is essentially an outpatient. These two practice settings, hospital and ambulatory care, require different nursing skills; that is, in each setting, nurses have a specific set of role behaviors.

The concept of groups and families with its members functioning within a system is not necessarily new. The content of this section of the book provides the answers to such questions as: What constitutes a family support system? Who are the members that make up the system?

Nurses communicate in a variety of professional settings, role relationships, and contexts. As their professional role continues to expand, nurses are beginning to lead groups and work with families in increasing numbers.

There are numerous types of groups in which nurses can be either a leader or a member. These groups have formed essentially to provide mutual support for the client members of the group. Interactions among the group members can be complex. Thus, working with groups and families can be fraught with difficulties, many of which are centered around communication. Members of the group, as well as the family of the client, also have special needs relating to their feelings.

In the following two chapters, communication in the hospital and ambulatory settings is discussed as well as how clients use certain communication patterns within a group or family system.

Communication in the Hospital and Ambulatory Settings

BEHAVIORAL OBJECTIVES

By reading this chapter and participating in its exercises, students will be able to:

1. Describe five nurse–client communication barriers in hospital nursing practice settings
2. Explain the characteristics of a bureaucracy
3. Distinguish between team and primary nursing staffing patterns
4. Understand how the concepts of space, multidirectional communication, multichannel communication, and triadic communication affect communication patterns
5. Discuss the relationship between ambulatory care settings and primary care nursing
6. Describe the role of the nurse as information and information giver
7. Recognize three barriers to effective communication by primary care nurses in their roles as information takers

---

COMMUNICATION IN THE HOSPITAL SETTING

Communication in the hospital setting can be examined from three viewpoints: the physical setting, the organization of activities within the setting, and communication concepts specific to the hospital setting.

THE PHYSICAL SETTING

Physical setting refers to the impact of the layout and design of rooms, furniture, lighting, and other aspects of what is usually called the physical environment, as well as the types of medical equipment used and the ways in which communication is carried out. Often, the physical setting of the hospital itself contributes to clients' reluctance to express feelings. Clients are anxious; they are physically and, to some extent emotionally, dependent. They may perceive themselves as being in a hostile environment. These reactions are frequently the result of communication barriers that can be present in any hospital setting. Five such barriers are:

1. The use of technical language
2. Noise level
3. The rigid routine
4. "Busy" atmosphere
5. Uniforms

The Use of Technical Language. The use of technical language inhibits the communication process. Hospital personnel who are accustomed to the clinical setting often forget that many clients do not understand medical terminology as well as "in-house" jargon. Examples such as "Mrs. Thompson is due for her p.o. med. stat!" or "Did you send Mrs. Thomas's cath spec to the lab?" are often spoken in the presence of the client. An example taken from a diary kept by a female surgical client who was hospitalized for a possible mastectomy shows the confusion that can occur with the use of technical language.

> It's already hard to remember what the world was like before hospital rounds. . . . They came and stood around and the leader poked around on me and said, "That's a fibroma." I never heard the word before but I know what the ending means—sarcoma, carcinoma—O God! He didn't say it to me, he never talked to me at all, but he said it to the others. . . . All I'm doing is sitting here crying and shaking and smoking and listening to that word echoing around inside my head (Roberts, C., 1977, p. 51).

Some 24 hours later, after surgery, which had not necessitated mastectomy, the client discovered that despite its sound, the word "fibroma" did not indicate malignancy. She continued to feel, however, that the doctor had been in error to have spoken in her presence without explaining to her what it meant. Her final comment on the subject was "It's hard to forgive 12 hours of terror that needn't have happened at all."

Some guidelines to use when talking to clients in the hospital are:

- Use language clients can understand.
- When it is necessary to use hospital terms, explain to client.
- Key the explanation to the intellectual level of the client.
- Watch clients who are "first admissions."
- Ask for feedback.
- Guard against use of "hospital jargon" with coworkers within hearing of clients.

Noise Level. Despite signs to the contrary, the hospital is a noisy place. Many people go in and out of rooms with carts, charts, medications, and meals. It may be difficult to find a quiet place to talk privately to a client. One area where the noise level tends to present a problem is in critical care.

In spite of the intermittent loud noises or the constant high level of noise from machines and suctioning equipment, the most disturbing auditory stimuli according to clients recalling their experiences were *staff communications!* (Noble, 1979). Staff, especially nurses and physicians, in order to overcome the noise factor within the acute care environment, raise their voices and are often within earshot of the client.

Rigid Routine. Clients are overtly and subtly encouraged to conform to the hospital environment. In some hospitals, if baths are given in the A.M., the client receives the bath in the A.M., whether or not he or she feels it is needed. Meals, naps, temperatures, other procedures and doctors' visits can be routinized in the hospital environment. Clients often feel it is necessary to conform to routinized and sanctioned "times to talk" and may become "good patients" if it is not the "correct time to share," such as when the nurse is tending to another client in the same room.

"Busy" Atmosphere. The majority of hospital settings are characterized by activity and movement. The larger the hospital, the more this is apparent. The hospital setting with a high degree of activity and "busy" atmosphere can influence nurse–client communication. The "hustle and bustle" atmosphere of the average hospital setting does not lend itself readily to effective and meaningful communication between clients, nurses, and other

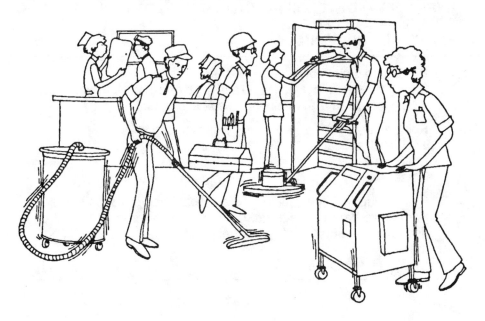

health professionals. At times, clients feel that there is a sense of urgency in what nurses are doing and that their own concerns are too small to be important. They do not want to take up the nurses' valuable time talking about feelings. Some of the most effective communication occurs during the evening and night shifts when there are fewer health professionals present and a more relaxed atmosphere prevails.

Similarly, nurses may feel that they are too busy to take the time to give therapeutic care. This may be due to task realities, the nurse's own discomfort talking to clients, or a sense that this is not "the right place" to spend time talking. The nurse who continually senses this is "not the right time" has allowed the "busy" atmosphere to interfere with effective nurse–client communication.

Uniforms. A major purpose of the uniform is to identify staff position to the client; it also identifies a nurse's position to other staff within the hospital. The traditional white dress and cap is not often seen in the hospital. One reason for this is that it has been identified with nurses in subordinate roles in the media, which has created a negative image. A second reason is that darker colors, as well as skirted or vested suits are perceived as more powerful, whereas a white uniform can diminish one's perceived power (Lamar, 1985). Nurses tend to wear uniforms that identify their specific work area, such as scrubs in the ICU or lab coats over a white skirt with no cap on a general unit. This can be a communication barrier to the patient who has difficulty distinguishing LPNs from RNs and female physicians. A pin with name and title often serves as the most accurate means of identification.

EXERCISE IN DEVELOPING STRATEGIES TO HANDLE COMMUNICATION BARRIERS IN THE HOSPITAL ENVIRONMENT

1. Divide into groups of three.
2. Each group will either pick or be assigned one of the following communication "barriers" within the hospital milieu:

Roommates	Busy atmosphere
Technical language	Change of routing in different
Uniforms	shifts
Noise level	Fragmented nursing care

3. Each group will then think of one additional barrier *not* on the list.
4. For its two barriers, each group will come up with three ways of decreasing the impact of the barrier on effective nurse–client communication.
5. Share your strategies.

Organization of Activities Within the Setting

The organization of activities in a hospital setting is bureaucratic. A bureaucracy has four major characteristics (Tappan, 1983):

1. Division of labor: In the hospital there is a clear division of labor, and activities are distributed among members who perform or are responsible for only those tasks they are assigned.
2. Hierarchy of authority: All positions are arranged in a hierarchy. There are designated superior and subordinate positions; the superior initiates the action and the subordinate is the recipient of action. Each person is held accountable to a superior.
3. Rules and regulations: There are standard operating procedures that define and regulate all behavior, for example, policy manuals and procedure books.
4. Emphasis on technical competence: People with certain skills and knowledge are hired to carry out specific parts of the total work of the organization.

Bureaucracies are closed systems; they do not easily adapt to change. Bureaucratic hospitals are supposedly models of efficiency in that many tasks are accomplished, but what is gained in being efficient may be lost in poor communication patterns. The four major attributes of a bureaucracy affect nursing communication in the following ways:

Division of Labor.   There is much contact with other health professionals in the hospital setting yet there is little or no communication among health professionals representing various clinical subspecialties at a departmental or interdepartmental level. Nurses communicate primarily with other nurses; physicians share a greater sense of collegiality with other physicians than with professionals from other fields. The high level of specialization present in the hospital encourages little or no communication among subspecialties of these professions. That is, operating room nurses communicate primarily with other operating room nurses, and pediatric nurses tend to communicate with other pediatric nurses.

Interdepartmental communication is often a problem in the bureaucratic structure of the hospital. Other departments do not have the same set of priorities as the floor unit. For example, a nurse calls the surgical supply department to order a tracheostomy set and is told by the receiver of the call that the old set must be returned before a new one can be sent to the floor. The nurse's top priority is to get the tracheostomy set as soon as possible because of a crisis situation; the technician in the surgical supply department has different priorities, ones given by the supervisor.

Division of labor encourages written memos and directives on printed forms, that is, one-way communication with no opportunity for the receiver to provide immediate feedback. Person-to-person contact is limited, leading to a sense of isolation and alienation of individuals working or receiving nursing care in the system.

Hierarchy of Authority. A bureaucracy implies levels of authority in which one is responsible to a superior but at the same time has control over a subordinate. Downward communication often centers around direction giving in relation to job role, hospital policies, or rules. Upward communication tends to keep the person who is in the one-up position attuned to what is going on in the bureaucracy. Upward communication needs to be encouraged, as downward communication is easier than upward communication. "Open door policies" and/or frequently scheduled meetings between supervisors and staff encourages upward communication and are essential for mutual decision making in a hierarchical hospital setting.

Hierarchy of authority is present in team nursing while primary nursing promotes horizontal communication between members of the nursing team. In team nursing, the nursing staff (RNs, LPNs, nursing assistants, and aides) is divided into teams and each team is assigned to a specific location in the hospital. The team is responsible for a designated group of clients. Acutely ill clients are usually assigned to the most capable and experienced members of the team. The team leader assigns the duties to the team members on an *ad hoc* basis during each shift and reports directly to the head nurse. There is a clear hierarchy of authority. Communication follows the same lines. The team leaders report to the head nurse, who reports to the supervisor, who reports to an assistant or the director of nursing. The team leader can also communicate "down" to the RN on the team, who communicates to the LPN, who communicates to an aide.

Team nursing places the nurse in a "middle management" position; one in which the nurse is giving and receiving communication from both "above" and "below." When messages conflict, highly stressful situations result. The team leader may find him- or herself in a "double-bind" position of receiving conflicting messages from above and below as in the following example.

Head Nurse (to team leader): Ambulate Mr. Jones today.
Team Leader (to staff nurse): Ambulate Mr. Jones.
Staff Nurse (to team leader): Mr. Jones will not get out of bed. He is threatening to call his doctor if the nurses do not leave him alone.

While the first priority is the client, who is at the bottom of the hierarchy, there is a natural inclination to obey orders from above.

The primary nurse assumes 24-hour responsibility for a limited number of clients (four to six). Clients are assigned to a primary nurse until they are discharged or transferred, and he or she directs the overall care of the client on a 24-hour basis through orders that are written on the care plan, as well as through other channels of communication when the nurse is not on duty. The primary nurse has the authority and autonomy to plan and implement care. He or she communicates directly with the physician and the client. The head nurse serves as a resource consultant to all nurses concerning problems in client care.

The advantages of primary nursing in facilitating communication are obvious. By having total responsibility, the nurse can focus on emotional as well as physical needs when they arise. The nurse also serves as a direct link to the client at all times. In one study, clients who had a primary nurse perceived that their care was delivered by technically and professionally competent nursing staff, that the primary nurses kept them informed about what was happening to them and gave them a chance to talk about their problems and that their nursing care included a trusting relationship between themselves and the nurses caring for them (McClelland et al., 1987). Second-generation primary nursing is case management and is based on the premise that nursing service is an individualized set of outcomes for each patient. The primary nurse is a manager of a caseload of patients (Zander, 1985).

Rules and Regulations. Rules and policies in a hospital setting tend to foster rigidity, creating communication barriers as well as enforcing a closed system. There are standard procedures for all nursing behaviors, and these discourage suggestions or creativity from outside sources. Most nursing systems have explicit written procedures to insure client safety and cost effectiveness within the hospital. Gross violation fo rules and procedures in the hospital could be threatening to client care. At the same time, these rules and procedures contribute to overly rigid boundaries.

Emphasis on Technical Competence. The fourth characteristic of a bureaucracy is an impersonal attitude. There is a tendency in a bureaucratic system, such as a hospital organization, to place a higher value on the high-visibility psychomotor aspects of nursing than on the cognitive-thinking or the affective-feeling aspects of nursing. In other words, the nurse who is task-oriented as opposed to the nurse who is more person-oriented is more highly rewarded for visible accomplishments. It should be emphasized here that some nurses may rate high on person orientation; others may rate high on task orientation; and some may rate high or low on both; in other words, it has been determined that person and task orientations are not either/or but may be found in various combinations in different individuals (McFarland et al., 1984).

Communication Concepts Specific to the Hospital Setting. At this point, the complexity of communication within the bureaucratic hospital setting has become obvious. There are four concepts that are useful in examining how blocks and miscommunication occur in the hospital setting: space, multidirectional communication, multichannel communication, and triadic communication.

The Concept of Space.   The concept of space implies the distance one feels comfortable in interactions with others. There are two dimensions to this concept: physical space and a sense of space in the abstract sense, referred to as personal space.

Physical space can directly influence the pattern and level of communication interaction in a nurse–client dyad. For example, if a client wishes to share feelings of anxiety with a nurse and finds him- or herself in a four-bed unit where roommates can overhear, he or she will not be able to share fears and anxieties easily. Nurses who are effective in nurse–client communication have developed a sense of respect for the client's sense of physical space. Knocking before entering the client's room, standing at the foot of the bed while talking to the client, and calling the client by name are ways of giving the client a sense of territory and more physical space.

Personal space is defined as an area with invisible boundaries into which another person, in this case the nurse, is not welcome. Personal space has

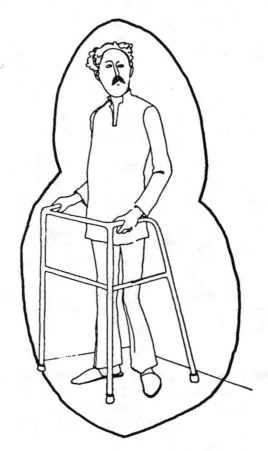

been referred to as a "bubble" that surrounds an individual. The size of the bubble can vary depending on several factors. One factor is familiarity, that is, the degree to which two persons are familiar with one another or the attitudes they have toward one another. Persons who know each other will exhibit smaller personal space zones than those who are strangers.

One's sense of personal space is usually reflected in the distance one attempts to maintain from the other person. The more one perceives the other's status as higher or one-up, the greater the distance between them (Lamar, 1985). This is also apparent in ethnic differences in personal space as well. For example, white Americans require greater space than Europeans who in turn require greater space than South Americans.

A final factor that influences one's sense of personal space is the nature of the transaction. In nurse–client interactions, the fact that the client is in the hospital and the nurse is overseeing his or her care legitimizes the nurse's "invasion" of the client's bubble. Personal space is violated repeatedly in acute illness states because of the need for nursing interventions such as giving injections, insertion of intravenous lines, and the use of monitoring devices. These numerous violations of personal space by nurses and other coworkers, especially in such instances where they do not take the time to introduce themselves or explain their purpose, often lead to heightened anxiety on the part of the client.

Nurses, as well as clients, prefer a sense of territory in which they can feel secure. Often, the restrictive physical dimensions of a nurses' station prohibit a sense of territory. The nurse's territory is often reduced to a locker in a cloakroom or perhaps to a small cubicle where group meetings are held. There is no desk or physical space that nurses can identify as their "turf" nor is there an easily accessible private place ("privacy retreat") the nurse can go to for quiet and relaxation.

A vital strategy for survival is solitude, a time to be with oneself and attain a positive state of being. There is little encouragement in the hospital setting to engage in solitude seeking behavior. Much of the stress, irritability, and fatigue of nurses might be attributed to the fact that their privacy is almost continuously invaded by clients, physicians, and other nurses during an 8-hour period. Certainly, nursing lounges near the units in which they are working would help to serve the need for nurses' privacy retreat.

Multidirectional Communication. Communication in the hospital setting is multidirectional. That is, nurses can communicate downward, upward, and horizontally.

Downward Communication. Most communication flow between nurses in the hospital is higher to lower levels. This is because there is a need for superiors to convey a great deal of information; in other words, nurses working in hospitals see less need to receive information from others and more need to send information than do people in other organizational contexts.

Downward communication flow accomplishes several purposes: to give specific task directives about job instructions; to give information about organizational procedures and practices; and to tell subordinates about their performance (Rakich, Beaufort, & O'Donovan, 1977). Unfortunately, few, if any downward communication interactions are designed so that subordinates can talk and superiors listen, such as requests for information and opinions. Some helpful ways to improve downward communication are:

1. Know yourself. Subordinates can know more about you than you do. Listen to what nurses are trying to tell you about yourself in terms of which order gets the fastest reaction. Subordinates usually know what is important to you, in order to survive the stresses of their jobs.
2. Be aware of your nonverbal behavior. It has already been stated that words constitute only 7% of the total message. Nonverbal gestures such as body lean and posture and tone of voice can be more important than what you are saying to a nurse who is in a subordinate position.
3. Take time to listen in order to obtain feedback. Often this is the most effective way to find out what is going on within your unit.

Upward Communication. Upward communication in most hospital settings is characteristically described as "poor" and "few in number." Upward communication provides nurse managers or nurses in authority with decision-making information, reveals problem areas, provides data for performance evaluation, and indicates the status of worker morale. Unfortunately, the higher the communication goes, the more garbled and greater the chance of total elimination of the message.

Lateral or Horizontal Communication. Nurses feel more comfortable talking with each other rather than communicating with nurses in superior or inferior positions. One explanation for this tendency is that the culture of nursing has not encouraged communication about problems. Nurses are expected to complete assignments and to be able to look up answers if they do not know them. The reluctance to communicate with superiors has been attributed to time pressures. Lateral communication can be informal; this type of communication flow is often called "the grapevine" or "rumor." Characteristics of the grapevine are that it is fast, selective, and discriminating as to who hears what from whom, and tends to be jointly active with formal lines of communication. Informal communication can be used effectively for transmission of information, especially if one wants the message to get distributed in a hurry! It tends to be distributed in a cluster-like fashion rather than a straight chain in which A tells B, who then tells C, who then tells D, and so on. Research shows that the grapevine follows a cluster chain pattern: A tells three or four others (B, C, and D). One of these will tell three or four others, and so on. As the information becomes older, and the proportion of those knowing gets larger, it gradually dies out, because those who know it do not repeat it (Rakich, Beaufort & O'Donovan, 1977).

Multichannel Communication. The simultaneous use of more than one channel is necessary in order for the nurse to respond adequately to the hospital environment. Many events, the majority of which are stressful, are occurring at the same time. The frenetic pace of the floor or hospital wing is obvious. When nurses go from busy hallways into quiet interiors of acutely ill clients' rooms, they are required to shift gears and readjust communication behavior, as well as their level of cognition. When seeking information from clients, nurses must initiate the communication process by briefly encapsulating what is being asked and why. Clients do not possess the shorthand skills that nurses have, and this mandates that nurses must be explicit when seeking information from clients.

It is important for students and new staff to recognize that becoming more adept at sorting out multisource messages depends on nurses' becoming more familiar with their role. Clients do not have this familiarity with the setting. Because of this, they are often "paced" by the multistimuli environment; that is, they let the pace of the events affect their communication behavior.

> When the nurse went to give Mr. Johnson his A.M. care, he (Mr. Johnson) was visibly upset over the disappearance of his pajama bottoms. The nurse looked everywhere in his bedside unit and immediately reported the loss to her team leader, who informed the head nurse. After the head nurse called the laundry and no pajama bottoms were found, the problem started to escalate until the entire staff was either commenting on Mr. Johnson's loss or actively looking for the bottoms. Finally, Mrs. Brown, an instructor for the nursing students, came to the floor, entered Mr. Johnson's room and asked, "When was the last time you saw the pajama bottoms?" Mr. Johnson replied, "When the night nurse removed them because I perspired with a high fever."
>
> Mrs. Brown, thinking that perhaps the night nurse might have rinsed them out, looked in the bathroom adjoining Mr. Johnson's unit and found the bottoms drying on a towel rack.

The nurse (and others) in this situation let the client's anxiety put them into a high state of activity rather than attempting to solve the problem at a more appropriate pace.

Oftentimes communication problems arise due to timing as well as pacing:

> Mrs. Hayes, a 70-year-old diabetic, had doctor's orders to have her 7 A.M. insulin after she had eaten her breakfast. The aide told the medication

nurse that Mrs. Hayes had eaten and her tray was removed. The aide also gave the same information to the student assigned to Mrs. Hayes. The medication nurse prepared the insulin and gave it to Mrs. Hayes. She did not record it immediately on the chart or kardex. Within 5 minutes the student nurse prepared the *second* insulin injection and, under the supervision of her instructor, administered the injection.

Simultaneous messages in the above situation created a serious error. The error was created because of lack of communication in the following ways:

- The aide informed two nurses, both of whom assumed they would be the one to give the medication without checking with each other.
- The medication nurse did not record the medication immediately.
- The client did not inform the student she had already had the injection.

Triadic Communication

A doctor and a nurse are talking to each other in a client's room in the hospital. The client had a hernia operation and the doctor is questioning the nurse about the client with reference to her order, "Ambulate twice a day." The client is listening to the conversation between the doctor and the nurse, shifting her eyes from one to the other as they converse. How many people are there in this conversation?

Up to this point, dyadic communication has been the basis for discussion of communication interactions. Dyadic communication involves two people in a face-to-face interaction. Many communication interactions involve more than two people, however, and are referred to as triadic communication. A triad is a social system composed of three people transacting in a face-to-face situation (Wilmot, 1975). Many forms of triadic communication exist in nursing. If one were to analyze the communication interaction between nurse and physician, as in the above situation, one could conclude that the majority of nurse–physician interactions are essentially *about* the client. The client might be present during the interaction (as in this situation). Thus, the client becomes a third member in the interaction even though nothing is contributed to the communication by him or her. She functioned in the above example as a listener.

Interactions that are three-way, as in Figure 9–1, have tendencies to cause the formation of coalitions; that is, two members will pair up in opposition to the third. Even more revealing is the fact that these coalitions can be predicted with considerable accuracy if the relative power of the three members

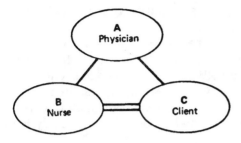

Figure 9–1. A communication triad with *B* (nurse) and *C* (client) forming a coalition against *A* (physician).

is known (Caplow, 1968). In this situation, it can be predicted that the nurse (*B*) will probably form a coalition with the client (*C*), depending on the amount of authority that the physician (*A*) chooses to use. If *A* is threatening, *B* and *C* will become mutually supportive of each other in order to protect themselves against the superior authority of *A*. While this is not the outcome in every situation of this type, a tendency toward the coalition of *B* and *C* is often felt in situations such as the one presented, and the *B* and *C* coalition should result more frequently than by chance alone.

Consider the following situation:

A nurse is in Mrs. Scott's room performing health teaching with a client who is going to have a cardiac catherization. The client has told the nurse that she knows nothing about what is going to happen to her. The client's doctor enters the room, observes what is going on and turns to the client and says, "I will perform your catherization tomorrow. I've done many of these procedures before, so don't worry about it."

He turns to the nurse and says, "Have Mrs. Scott ready at 10 A.M." and leaves the room.

In this situation, the physician's use of authority has increased the affiliation of nurse and client. They both feel a sense of helplessness due to the physician's approach and they may join forces for mutual support. Contrast this with an approach on the part of the physician in which he addresses the nurse by name and acknowledges the teaching she is providing the client and also addresses the client, asking if there is anything she does not understand. The tendency towards a coalition between the client and nurse is considerably lessened, and all three parties are more likely to have open communication with each other.

Triads are omnipresent in the hospital health care setting. The above situation could be replicated by using a head nurse (*A*), a staff nurse (*B*), and a client (*C*) or a staff nurse (*A*), an aide (*B*), and a client (*C*). Staff nurses have more authority than aides, who have more authority than clients. Are there situations in which the aide forms a coalition with the client to counteract the authority of the staff nurse? An experienced staff nurse could undoubtedly cite many situations.

In nurse–client–family member triads, the tendency toward the formation of a coalition between the family member and the client is often seen. One area around which the interaction between the families of clients and nurses in the hospital setting can revolve is visiting hours. In nurse–client–family member triads, nurses have the ultimate control and power; they often find themselves functioning as "gatekeeper" over the family for the visiting hour period.

The most important technique that the nurse can utilize in family–nurse communication is the use of empathy. It is not always easy to place oneself in the other person's frame of reference, especially when one's actions are subject to misinterpretation. Keeping the family member informed at all times as to exactly what is happening will alleviate stress and anxiety.

COMMUNICATION IN THE AMBULATORY CARE SETTING

Ambulatory care settings are traditionally located outside the hospital. Such settings include outpatient clinics, health maintenance organizations (HMOs), physicians' offices, schools, industries, or the client's home. Ambulatory care nursing can encompass the total management of chronic illness as well as provide for health maintenance and health promotion. Health care directed toward clients who are well or in the nonacute stages of illness in an ambulatory care setting is referred to as *primary care*. This term is not to be confused with primary nursing even though the philosophy inherent in primary nursing is similar to that of primary care (Stanhope & Lancaster, 1988).

Primary care givers have authority, autonomy, and accountability. *Primary care* usually implies the context in which the client's initial contact with the health care system takes place; also, it can imply continued surveillance of a chronic illness state in which the client's contact with the system is more sporadic, where clients are in and out of the system.

Consultative and referral resources are less readily available in these settings than in an acute care setting. Primary care nurses utilize assessment skills often. They also act as coordinators for *all* health services, setting priorities in order to meet the client's needs. Primary care nurses use innovative and less standardized means of meeting the health needs of clients— health needs which are usually less predictable and require monitoring over a long period of time.

Primary care represents the nursing mode of the future. The emphasis in health care from illness to wellness has shifted much of nursing's focus from caring for clients to diagnosing and treating responses to illness and health problems and client teaching. Many of the health problems today can be brought on by environmental factors, such as lung cancer's relationship to smoking, and chronic heart disease influenced by diet and lifestyle. The incidence of these chronic disease conditions will disappear only over an extended period of time. Solutions will not come overnight. The answers to these chronic conditions will constitute one focus of nursing in the future.

Greater emphasis is placed on the nurse's role in the management of chronic illness in the community setting rather than on the nurse's role in health maintenance in a clinical setting such as a community health clinic. This is because students are more likely to have experiences in community health settings; although many will spend time in health clinics. Both roles have been included in this chapter. One goal of this chapter is to familiarize the student with the role of the nurse in the ambulatory care setting in order to provide a foundation for future learning. The chapter covers communication between the client and the nurse in the ambulatory care setting and discusses some of the barriers that exist in nurse–client interactions in this setting.

Communicating in the Home Care Setting

A major segment of ambulatory nursing practice is in the home care setting. Look at the following situation:

> Mr. Booth is a 75-year-old widower who lives alone. His sole income is from Social Security. Mr. Booth has diabetes complicated by peripheral vascular disease. His visual acuity is poor. The VNA nurse is making a home visit in order to change the dressing on an ulcerated area on Mr. Booth's leg. Mr. Booth feels lonely and isolated, and his knowledge of community resources is limited.

One trend in primary care nursing is for persons with varying degrees of illness and disability to be cared for in their homes. Nurses are frequently called on to make home visits, assess the living environment, and administer care to individuals who have been in the hospital or are in need of their services. There are several issues that make communication in the home different from hospital or clinic settings. The first is that interviews and care are given on the client's "territory," rather than on the nurse's. This means that clients may feel that their personal environment is being invaded or, conversely, that they have more power and control over their care than in the hospital setting.

A related issue is the sense that the client is the "host" for the nurse. It is important to respect this positive role, especially with minority group members, and show appropriate responses like accepting a cup of tea or letting the client do something for the nurse.

Also, there are likely to be more distractions (radios, telephone calls, visitors) that the nurse cannot easily control. There may be a need to limit these intrusions during an important visit. Similarly, these "intrusions" may also give excellent information about the client's relationships with family, friends, and other parts of the support system.

Finally, the home visit is an excellent opportunity to gather indirect information about the safety, logistics, and other environmental aspects of the home, including cleanliness. The nurse can make specific suggestions and see if they are implemented on subsequent visits. If instructions need to be written down, there is the opportunity to ensure that they are posted where they can be seen. Although some nurses feel uncomfortable going into another person's home to administer treatment, the opportunities and necessities for home care make communicating and treating the client in the home a growing concern for the nursing profession.

The client, especially in the home care setting, is not usually seen as a single individual; rather he or she is viewed within the family context. Thus, in the home setting, the nurse is exposed to family members as well as the client.

Guidelines for communicating with clients in their homes include:

1. Pay attention to physical surroundings. Be sure that distractions, such as radio and television, are minimized.
2. If you need time with the client to review a procedure or discuss an important concern, ask family members for privacy.
3. You may be required to move chairs or other furniture in order to communicate directly. Ask permission to do so, recognizing that this is the client's turf.

The Nurse in the Ambulatory Care Setting

In any ambulatory care setting, the nurse functions both as an information taker and an information giver. Some essential tasks of primary care nurses involve the dual functions of eliciting information *from* the client and imparting information *to* the client. A discussion of each of the functions follows:

Primary Care Nurses as Information Takers. The use of information-gathering skills is an essential part of the primary care nurse's role. The communication tool for information-gathering is the interview (Chapter 5), which may be structured or unstructured. Incorporated within the structured interview is the nursing history, which is often used by primary care nurses in outpatient settings. Nonstructured interviews are more often undertaken by the nurse in the client's home setting. In order for nurses to formulate nursing diagnoses, they must use effective information-gathering skills, and also be aware of the pitfalls in interviewing. It is important that nurses understand the nature of interpersonal techniques used in interviewing clients, in order to increase their ability to utilize congruent responses.

Oftentimes, primary care nurses lack certain pieces of information about a client. There is no chart readily at hand, such as in the hospital. Nurses are apt to have only half the essential information needed and must piece together the rest, either by consulting another health professional or by talking to the client. One piece of information that is not always available is the client's previous contacts with the health care system. Previous negative experiences in the health care system will impact on the present nurse–client interaction. Obviously, if a client has had a contact with a nurse who made no attempt to understand the client and the client felt put down, the next contact will be affected even though it is not with the same nurse. The client does not wish to be subjected to the same negative experience and will withhold trust.

Primary Care Nurses as Information Givers. In assuming the role of a teacher, the nurse must start where the client is. It is unrealistic, for example, to teach a client to administer his or her own insulin injections if the client's hands are somewhat crippled with arthritis. If the nurse's objective is to teach a young mother about the importance of immunization shots for her baby, the feasibility of the mother's being able to obtain the shots must be considered. Does the mother have to take a taxi across town and then wait for 2 hours in the outpatient clinic? The goal of the nurse is to give the client a sense of "want to do." Coercion does not work because the nurse is not always there. Clients must be internally motivated and able to perceive the health problem in order to carry out their own effective health care.

Both client and nurse have their own interpersonal style in the teaching situation. They bring to the situation their own internalized frames of reference. Nurses generally have an unchanging communication style. Thus, if a nurse tends to be a nondirective listener, she or he will probably use that communication style in every client situation. Some nurses have been identified as "client-focused," that is, they pick up the clients' cues; and others are "nurse-focused," that is, they respond to their own frame of reference.

In their role as information givers or teachers, nurses will often see clients who attempt to place a single causality on all health-related problems. The tendency to relate illness to one cause is called linear thinking. Examples of linear thinking are:

- I caught this cold because my feet got wet.
- My cancer was due to all that stress.

In actuality the cold might have been due to a number of factors: fatigue, lowered resistance, or exposure to others. The cancer also might have been influenced by more than one variable: a history of cancer in the family, repeated exposure to carcinogens in the environment, or age-related factors. The temptation is to say $A(\text{cause}) = X(\text{illness})$, to attach a single variable to the cause of illness. Illness is usually multicausal: $A + B + C + D = X$. All the factors combined lead to the disease (X).

Clients often punish themselves by attributing their health problems to a single cause. In these instances, the nurse, through use of therapeutic communication, may have to reestablish the client's former sense of self-worth and change the client's patterns of thinking. If linear thinking is preventing the client from undertaking the proper health regimen, then the nurse must reinforce more complex thinking as opposed to linear explanations.

CONCLUSION

A system of hospital nursing practice can be described in relation to the physical setting, organization of activities, and four communication concepts specific to the hospital setting: space, mutidirectional communication, multi-channel communication, and triadic communication. Nurses who practice in these settings have the opportunity to relate the concepts presented here to their interactions with clients and other staff.

An additional focus is on the nurse's role in ambulatory care nursing practice and how the role influences communication. The nurse in the ambulatory care setting has a dual role of eliciting information *from* the client and imparting information *to* the client. In many instances, the nurse and client can actually switch roles, allowing the nurse to be the learner and the client the teacher. This is particularly true in nurse–client situations in which the client represents a different ethnic group and culture.

Primary care nursing provides an exciting challenge to nurses who choose to work in this setting. The nursing role is associated with greater autonomy and more independent decision making. Effective communication skills assume a large part of this role.

REFERENCES

Caplow, T. *Two against one coalition in triads.* Englewood Cliffs, N.J.: Prentice-Hall, 1968.

Lamar, E. K. Communicating personal power through nonverbal behavior. *Journal of Nursing Administration*, 1985, 15(1), 41–44.

McClelland, M. R., Kolesar, M. J., & Bailey, M. A. From team to primary nursing. *Nursing Management*, 1987 18(10), 69–71.

McFarland, G. K., Leonard, H. S., & Morris, M. M. *Nursing leadership and management.* New York: John Wiley & Sons, 1984.

Noble, M. A. Communication in the ICU: Therapeutic or disturbing? *Nursing Outlook*, 1979, 27, 195–198.

Rakich, J. S., Beaufort, B., & O'Donovan, T. R. *Managing health care organizations.* Hinsdale, Ill.: Dryden Press, 1977.

Roberts, C. *Doctor and patient in the teaching hospital: A tale of two life-worlds.* Lexington, Mass.: Lexington Books, 1977.

Stanhope, M., & Lancaster, J. *Community health nursing* (2nd ed.). St. Louis: C. V. Mosby Co., 1988.

Tappan, R. M. *Nursing leadership: Concepts and practice.* Philadelphia: F. A. Davis Co., 1983.

Wilmot, W. *Dyadic communication: A transactional perspective.* Reading, Mass.: Addison-Wesley, 1975.

Zander, K. Second generation primary nursing: A new agenda. *Journal of Nursing Administration,* 1985, 15(3), 18–24.

10 Communication with Groups and Families

BEHAVIORAL OBJECTIVES

By reading this chapter, students will be able to:

1. Discuss reasons for and against the use of group work
2. Describe common group dynamics and stages of group development
3. Describe parameters that affect group communication
4. Describe reasons for and barriers against communicating with families
5. List six guidelines that aid communication with families

References to group dynamics in nursing have traditionally emphasized such areas as interactions between the members of a group, the cohesiveness of the group, or the size of the group and its effect on group dynamics. In this chapter, the emphasis is on the nurse as a leader or facilitator of a group of clients. The material presented provides nurses with information on leading client groups; the psychosocial needs of clients are stressed.

A group is defined, for our purposes here, as two or more clients who are interdependent; they have a common task. The number of client groups that have emerged within the total health care system in recent years is staggering! Many of these groups have different tasks; some are therapeutic, for example, "stroke" groups or groups of diabetics or "ostomy" clients. Others are self-help groups, for example, Alcoholics Anonymous, Weight Watchers, and drug abuser groups. Still others are groups whose purpose is to promote growth and development or self-actualization. Examples are T-groups, encounter groups, or groups of elderly clients who are trying to become more assertive or to gain a healthier attitude about themselves through positive reminiscing.

Nurses are assuming much of the responsibility in health care settings in leading these groups. Communication in groups is one of the most complex, demanding, and yet often misunderstood areas for all health professionals. Why should this be true? What makes groups different from individuals? After all, communication patterns should be similar among individuals in terms of channels, styles, patterns, and goals, regardless if it takes place in a group setting.

The answers to these questions constitute the content of this chapter on group settings and communication. The nature of groups, their dynamics, and specific type of group and its goals, structural factors, the communication patterns characteristic of groups, the attributes of the leader, and the leader's function are the aspects that continually interact to affect the group's functioning (Shaw, 1980). It is the interaction of these factors that makes group work difficult yet exciting. These factors are outlined below.

Before each aspect of group functioning is discussed, a word of caution is given. The content presented on the following pages is intended to be an *introduction* to group work, as well as an examination of communication in groups. It is not intended to take the place of a course in group leadership, however, it can serve as a basis for further reading and learning about group process.

REASONS FOR GROUP WORK AND CAUTIONS TO CONSIDER

As was mentioned, nurses are moving toward group work in increasing numbers. A logical question to ask is "How come?" Why see a number of clients together rather than separately? There seems to be a variety of reasons nurses are choosing to do some of their work in a group context, as outlined in the following list:

- Cohesion—clients obtain a sense of identity (Yalom, 1985).
- Mutual emotional support—clients feel valued by peers.
- Therapeutic value of the group—certain issues and/or problems seem best handled in group setting.
- The group is a "laboratory" in which clients can learn about their own behavior in group settings and practice new behavior.
- Relationships—clients can develop meaningful relationships or make new friends.
- Interpersonal learning—clients can learn from each other.
- Options for participation—clients can have high or low participation and play a variety of "roles."
- Status—being in a group can be seen as high status by outsiders.
- Socialization.
- Cost-effectiveness—many clients can be worked with in a short period of time at a lower cost per client hour.
- Impact on systems—both the leader's visibility and the number of clients seen can have positive impact on the host system.

While all of these reasons are valid, some will not make sense in a given group setting. A nurse should consider using a group approach, however, whenever several of the reasons for doing so seem to fit the nursing context and the nurse has appropriate skills and supervision for the type of group (discussed below).

Cohesion.   Yalom (1985) defines cohesiveness as how attractive the group is to its members. While he does not feel that cohesion is in and of itself a "curative" process, he sees it as a precondition for therapy, and distinguishes between group and individual cohesiveness, the former roughly being an "addition" of all the individuals' sense of cohesiveness.

We consider the sense of cohesion slightly differently than Yalom, in part because we are writing about all of the kinds of group settings in which nurses might work. The sense of cohesiveness, that is, the sense of belonging or having an identity as a group member, is an important psychological asset. In our society, people obtain some pleasure from belonging to organizations, clubs, honor societies, colleges, and so on. At a *personal* level, group membership can be rewarding in and of itself, especially when the clients have few other positive social identifications, which can be the case for single parents, both institutionalized and community elderly, or adolescents. Thus, under the right circumstances, being a group member in and of itself will have value and can enhance the self-worth of the client.

Mutual Emotional Support.   Along with a sense of belonging, another advantage of the group is that members can provide emotional support for each other in ways the nurse cannot. For example, a nurse working with a group of diabetics will be seen as "not understanding how it is" unless the nurse, too, is a diabetic. Empathy may be more acceptable from a peer than from a health provider, both because peers know "how it is" (at least in the client's eyes) and because support may be easier to accept from an equal than from an "authority figure" such as a nurse.

Therapeutic Value of the Group.   The group experience carries with it the potential of being therapeutic (Yalom, 1985). That is, the experience of being in a group can help clients solve some of their own life problems, conflicts, and decisions by making a commitment and participating in group activities or sessions, depending on the goals of the group. In addition, some types of personal problems seem best handled in a group context, such as socialization or exchange of ideas. One notable example is Alcoholics Anonymous (the most effective treatment to date for alcoholism), which uses large group meetings as its work format.

The group is a laboratory in which clients can learn about their own behavior. Groups have both "real world" and "nonreal world" aspects. The real world aspect is that there are other people present who can observe the client and give their reactions and perceptions of the client's behavior, as well as giving emotional support. The nonreal world aspect of the group is that it is time-bound, has a nonwork focus, and a defined leader. These "laboratory" aspects mean that things that usually do not get communicated between people (like sharing observations about what each other just did and how it felt) can be emphasized and promoted by the group leader. Similarly, clients can try new behavior either in simulation (e.g., role playing with another client) or for real (e.g., making an explicit contract with other group members to use "I" statements for a session) in a context (the group) that is less risky than trying these things at home, on the job, or with friends. Thus, the group can become a relatively safe place to try new behavior before venturing out into the real world. The new behavior will still feel risky even in a safe and supportive group context.

Relationships. Group settings can provide the basis of personal relationships that can go beyond the time span of the group. A self-help group in a Senior Day Care Center, a group of coronary clients, or a health education group at a church can create or strengthen relationships between group members. This issue is quite important when the group is a major source of socialization for the clients (e.g., in a nursing home) and is time limited. In fact, the relationships may be more important than the work done by the leader!

Interpersonal Learning. A group setting offers group members the opportunity to learn from each other as well as receive emotional support. Depending on the focus of the group, clients' experience in dealing with the issues can provide useful options, (e.g., a nutrition group on ways to save money at the grocery store, or how to include exercise in a daily routine).

Options for Participation. In an individual setting, the client is expected to be an active participant in the communication process. In a group setting, there are opportunities to be a highly active participant, a moderately active participant, or even more of an observer. In addition, there are a variety of roles clients can take in group sessions, including gate-keeper, joker, leader's helper, voice of reason, passive, dominant, and others. While some may be more beneficial to the client and group than others, the opportunity to try new roles is a distinctive advantage of group settings.

Status. In certain settings, being a member of a group can be viewed as a sign of status. This has been observed in nursing homes and in senior citizen centers and is likely to take place in situations where the social environment is limited.

Socialization. A group setting can provide socialization for isolated individuals. Certain groups are designed specifically for this goal. In others, it is a byproduct.

Cost Effectiveness. Groups allow one nurse to be in contact with many clients at the same time. With an appropriate focus, the group setting costs less per client hour than individual sessions. Often, nurses who have to work with large numbers of clients who are geographically close and have shared psychosocial or health education problems will use groups for this reason.

Impact on Systems. The nurse who is running groups in an institutional setting becomes highly visible because of the need to schedule rooms and time for group meetings. Also, if clients are responding positively to the group experience, word can get out to that effect. This kind of notice and "good press" can have an impact on the host system, even if it is only noted by staff comments like "What are you doing?" The nurse who is interested in being an agent of change in the system could begin to use this success as a springboard to make changes, such as having staff groups around communication issues. A successful group or two can give the leader higher credibility in the system.

It should be noted that while each of the above reasons is an incentive for nurses to work with groups, it is rare that all of them will make sense in a specific setting. Similarly, there will usually be reasons for the nurse *not* to use group work. Several are listed below. The final decision on implementing a group approach will include a weighing of pros and cons, some assessment of the possibility of having groups in a particular setting, and a self-appraisal as to whether one has the prerequisite skills to undertake such a venture.

Cautions to Be Considered in Group Work

The following cautions should be viewed as concerns to be raised when groups are being considered. While the authors advocate the use of group methods by nurses, we feel that the educated nurse will also know the potential problems of group work and be able to minimize their impact on the group process.

- *The nurse may be unprepared or inadequately trained to work with the group.* There are no hard and fast guidelines for how to be prepared to work with groups. Different types of groups require different levels and types of skills from nurse leaders. For example, a health education class may require that the nurse know the cognitive material and be able to facilitate a discussion. On the other hand, working with a group of teenage drug abusers requires a knowledge of drugs, drug culture, and adolescent development, as well as skills in dealing with hostility, suspicion, low trust, low self-worth, and severe psychological problems.

  The usual ways in which the nurse receives experience in group work is to be a member of several types of groups (with acquaintances and/or friends), take some training in leading groups, and participate as a co-leader (or occasionally a leader) in a supervised setting. Even with appropriate background, it is always appropriate for the nurse to ask "Do I have the skills and knowledge necessary to run this particular group?" before taking on the responsibility of being a group leader.

- *The screening and selection processes for group membership can be inadequate.* George & Dustin (1988) present a thorough review of issues involved in screening clients for group experiences. There are several issues involved in deciding on group membership. Screening is considered to be an important aspect of group work for the group and the individual group members. The kinds of questions a nurse should ask before setting up a group include:

What is the purpose of the group? What are the characteristics of people who will benefit from the group?

What are the characteristics of potential members that will either not benefit or cause problems for other group members that would be detrimental to the group's goals?

How can I get information from prospective clients that ensures that the group members are likely to benefit from the experience?

How will clients be informed and give full consent to participate in the group?

By answering these questions in light of the type of group and situational context (hospital, community center, clinic, nursing home, day care center, etc.), the nurse should be able to come up with appropriate screening procedures (questionnaires, informed consent forms, interviews) for any group.

- *The heterogeneity of group members can leave some feeling left out; others may drop out.* Even with adequate screening, any group will represent a range of personalities, life styles, and health and emotional problems. Without careful monitoring by the leader, some clients may feel that the group is not for them, not verbalize it, and become passive members. Others may drop out, that is, attend infrequently or not at all.

  It may take personal contact via telephone or an individual interview to regain contact with a client who has dropped out of a group. This can be done as an "exit interview," which can be stipulated as a condition for joining the group.

- *Some group members can dominate at the expense of others: the most psychologically needy could take over.* This consideration is also related to certain group dynamics described below. Domination of "air time" in a group can be interpreted as the client's expression of a need for attention or control. If the focus of the group is on interpersonal relationships, then the leader can use the behavior as a source of group learning. If, however, the focus is on health problems, the exchange of ideas, or a focused group (weight loss, smoking, etc.), the "needy" person who dominates may have to be confronted or counseled out of the group setting, which requires a fair amount of assertion on the part of the nurse leader.

- *Some clients would derive more benefit from individual sessions.* One of the cautions in choosing group formats is that clients who can benefit from individual sessions may not receive the attention they need. These clients would include individuals who are not ready for a group setting or for whom the benefits of a group (cohesion, support) are not important in light of their health and psychosocial problems.

- *Some clients will be scapegoated.* One of the themes that can emerge in the life of a group is the scapegoating (blaming or putting down) of certain clients. The nurse has to be alert for scapegoating and must be able to provide some protection for the victim as well as have the skills required to use the process for the group's learning (if this fits the group's goals).
- *Negative status can be given to group members by others.* Although, as was mentioned earlier, positive status can be given to clients in certain group settings, it is just as easy for a negative status to be given to group membership by others, either out of ignorance, jealousy, or their own fears. Because the source of this labeling comes from outside the group, the nurse may only have indirect evidence, such as comments from staff in the halls before or after the group meetings. This is an issue that may have to be dealt with both at a group and organizational level.
- *A dependency relationship between the client and the nurse can develop and may not be worked through.* The issues of leadership are an integral part of group dynamics and are discussed later in this chapter. One precaution that goes with the power of being the leader is that clients may become dependent on the nurse as a source of validation of their behavior, feelings, and thoughts. While such dependency is an expected process in the life of many groups, it is important for nurses to be aware of the need for clients to work it through to the point where the nurse is no longer the powerful validating figure by the time the group's life is over. It is beyond the scope of this chapter to suggest how clients can be guided to work through dependency. The references at the end of this chapter provide further reading in this area.

GROUP DEVELOPMENT, PROCESSES, AND COMMUNICATION

In order to make sense out of the communication that takes place in groups, group leaders and researchers have developed several models for understanding *group development* and *group processes*. Group development means that the communication in groups varies in systematic ways or patterns throughout the group's life and that the systematic variations symbolize what can be called stages or phases of the group's life. Group processes (or group dynamics) refers to the implied relationships between group members at a moment in time in the group's life (Yalom, 1985). Group processes can be related to a series of conceptualizations or themes such as power and issues of leadership. Many of these themes are tied to stages of group development. As a way of introducing you to group processes, several major theories of group development are reviewed and group processes that occur in various stages are described, with examples of related communication.

One word of caution should be noted before launching into this subject. Group processes and development are difficult to unravel from immediate experience. That is, they are conceptualizations drawn out of a bewildering array of comments and gestures. (Think for a moment of all the things that go on in a classroom or seminar. Then try to distill the major underlying themes about how your group develops.)

The main theoretical frameworks that are commonly used to analyze group development are Bennis and Sheppard's (1956) stages of group development, Bion's (1961) concepts about "work-groups" and "basic assumption groups," the "focal conflict" model of group development (Whitaker & Lieberman, 1964), and Tuckman's phases of development (1965). There is significant overlap among these theories. A brief summary of each and a discussion of related dynamics follows.

Bennis and Sheppard's Model

Bennis and Sheppard (1956) suggested that there are two major issues that influence the development of any group, authority relationships (relations with the group leader) and personal relationships (relations among group members). They state that there are two general phases in the development of any group, the first phase being one of dependence (focusing on authority issues) and the second being interdependence (focusing on interpersonal issues). Each phase has its own subphases. In phase I, the subphases are submission, rebellion, and resolution of dependence. In phase II, the subphases are enchantment with member identification, disenchantment, and resolution of the interdependence problem. In addition, the movement between phases is uneven, with cycles of several steps forward, one backward, and so on.

One of the major contributions of this theory is to point out how different personalities in the group can be dominant at different stages of development. For example, if the group is in the counterdependent subphase (one of the subphases of dependency), it is expected that the people who are most counterdependent (either hostile to the leader or least tied emotionally to the leader) will exert the most influence.

Thus, in examining communication and influence of group members, the nurse should remember that at different times in the group's experience, various group members will be dominant. Also, dominance will shift as the group goes through different stages of development.

Bion's Concepts of "Basic Assumption" and "Work Groups"

As opposed to Bennis and Sheppard, Bion (1961) was less concerned with the sequence of group development than with the symbolic issues with which groups seem to deal. Bion made a distinction between two kinds of groups (or two basic stages of the same group). The key to the distinction is whether or not the group is dealing fully with the "real" issues at hand or is acting (communicating) as if an unspoken yet controlling assumption is determining how the group functions. This implies that the internal processes of the group take up its time and that it does not fully focus on "the task." The former group is called the "work group." The latter group is called a "basic assumption group." According to Bion, work groups are rare and usually come about after a group has "worked through" its basic assumption issues.

Bion posed three basic assumption groups: the dependency group, the fight–flight group, and the pairing group. The basic assumption of the dependency group is that the group is formed to receive security from the leader. The leader is supposed to protect the group member's comfort. The basic assumption of the fight–flight group is that the group meets to protect its members from the outside world. The choices are symbolic: whether to fight the world or flee. The pairing group meets with the basic assumption that it is to produce a savior, usually through a (symbolic) pairing of two group members.

The description of these three basic assumption groups may seem a little overdrawn. Remember, the three assumptions are conceptualizations that the group seems to be acting on, as deduced from what is communicated in the group. For example, on a given day, the group members may make comments like:

- Well, you're the leader, so you should take care of Bill.
- We can't hide anything from you!
- You're the only one who can do anything for us.

According to Bion's theory, these would indicate that the group is in a dependency state.

One could suspect that the group was acting in a fight–flight mode, if the statements being communicated were similar to:

- I don't trust any of this introspective stuff.
- I think everyone outside of this group thinks it's dumb.
- We should all get together and protest.

Finally, the expression of either hope or pairing suggests that the group is in a pairing phase if the communications could run along these lines:

- Things will improve when winter is over.
- Everyone ought to have marriage therapy.
- Bill and Sally here could really teach everyone a thing or two.

Bion's work has been used in many settings. It also includes guides for group leaders on how to help groups get through their assumption stages so they can become work groups. You are encouraged to read his book *Experiences in Groups* (1961) for a more indepth presentation of this material.

The Focal Conflict Model
Whitaker and Lieberman (1964) proposed a variation on the themes given in Bion's work to describe how therapeutic change takes place in groups,

although their concepts are useful in describing the dynamics of nontherapy groups as well. Their basic concepts include the following processes:

1. Individual behavior and communication in the group is collectively related to a singular unspoken concern about what is currently happening in the group.
2. All events that occur can be thought of as the expression of a hidden or covert conflict, which is the result of a wish that is opposed by a fear. Both parts are related to "here-and-now" issues.
3. When this "focal conflict" occurs, a solution is sought that will both satisfy the wish (as much as possible) and alleviate the fears.

What this simplified set of concepts implies is that the communication that goes on in groups can only be understood by trying to figure out the fear, the wish, and the "solution." All three have to be deduced from the overt communication.

As a simple example, consider the following statements that could be made by group members:

A: I'm tired. Maybe we could go home early tonight.
B: Me too, but weren't we told the sessions would last the full 2 hours?
C: Enough of this, let's get down to business.

Taking a focal conflict perspective, one could interpret A's statement as an expression of an underlying wish for independence (leaving early); B's agreement in being tired as a sign that the wish was shared; B's question about "being told" as a sign of fear or criticism by the leader; C's implied suggestion to drop the issue as a solution, and, if the others then changed the subject, acceptance of the solution. Obviously, the solution would be more direct if group members asked the leader about ending early, but in this group that "solution" would probably have been too threatening at that point. One would hope that the group would, over time, be able to deal with the independence issue through a series of "solutions" that become more and more direct.

Focal conflict theory is a useful set of concepts to use in understanding indirect communication in groups. It also alerts the leader to the fact that issues are continually being resolved and "re-resolved." Whitaker and Lieberman's book, *Psychotherapy Through the Group Process* (1964), explains the theory in detail.

Tuckman's Phases of Development

Tuckman (1965) proposed that groups go through four stages of development:

1. Forming
2. Storming

3. Norming
4. Performing

"Forming" refers to the initial interaction among group members and with the leader. There is a lot of initial testing of boundaries (limits of acceptable behavior), as well as the formation of dependency relationships with the leader.

Examples of communication that can be indicative of forming include:

- Will we meet for the full hour every week?
- Is it OK to smoke in here?
- Is anyone here married?

"Storming" refers to a stage of conflict and side-taking (polarization). Tempers may flare, and if the group has a defined task, it will be avoided or resisted. Examples of the kind of communication that is expected during the storming phase include:

- I think you're all picking on Jerry.
- Why do we have to do this, anyway?
- You're not listening to what I say!
- You three are all wrong. We just think alike, we're not against you.

In the "norming" stage, a sense of group cohesion occurs, there is some shift in roles as the group is no longer polarized, and new standards (or norms) for group communication emerge. It now may be possible to disagree without polarization or escalation of feelings:

- You know, I never thought I'd be able to say this to you, but I admire your brassiness.
- It seems like we disagree on this and that's OK.
- I'm tired of keeping peace. Someone else can do it.

The last stage Tuckman proposes is "performing." When a group is in a performing stage, it is able to use the resources of group members productively and creatively for the matter at hand. Group tasks can now be accomplished efficiently. Communication will focus more on task than on interpersonal or dynamic issues, although ideally, these issues will be dealt with openly if they arise.

The forming–storming–norming–performing sequence is easy to remember. It may also be a sequence that gets repeated in the same group over time, especially if a new member joins, the task is changed, or other factors significantly alter the group's life.

Other Aspects of Group Functioning That Affect Communication

Along with attending to the stage of the group's development, the group leader can also analyze the group's communication along the following dimensions (Corey et al., 1987; George & Dustin, 1988; Yalom, 1985).

Participation. Some group members will participate a great deal. Some will keep relatively quiet. Some members will help facilitate communication. Some will block it.

Styles of Influence. Styles of influence are related to styles of communication. Needless to say, the style (or "how") of influence will affect its impact. Four styles are (George & Dustin, 1988):

1. Autocratic—pushes to get own way
2. Peacemaker—avoids conflict, agrees
3. Laissez-faire—apparent lack of involvement
4. Democratic—tries to include everyone in decisions

Decision Making. How does the group make decisions? Some groups allow one member to make decisions unilaterally, without including others. Some groups vote. Some use consensus (all have to accept the solution, whereas in voting, all do not). In some groups, certain members make suggestions that have no impact, whereas other members' suggestions are implemented.

Task Functions. How does the group go about doing its task or solving a problem? Who gives feedback, who summarizes? Also, how does the group stay with the task as opposed to being tangential?

Morale Maintenance. Communication that is aimed at producing good working relationships among group members can be considered as serving the function of maintaining morale. This can be done by helping silent members participate (gate-keeping), stopping "over-talkers" (gate-closing), and supporting other group members' self-worth, even when there is disagreement with their ideas.

Group Atmosphere. The communication in a group will have a general feeling sense that is called group atmosphere. Groups can be friendly, warm, cool, intellectual, hostile, playful, and so forth. There may even be conflicting preferences in members' wishes for type of atmosphere.

Feedback. This dimension refers to how members verbalize approval, disapproval, criticism, and praise for each other.

Expression of Feelings. The whole question of how feelings are communicated in groups is an important one. Most of the feelings generated by group experience are not verbalized, especially in the early stages of the group's development. The leader has to look for visual and auditory cues for how members are feeling (e.g., body language, gestures, tone of voice).

Group Norms. Both what is communicated and what is not give clues as to what is acceptable behavior in the group. The rules of behavior may include which topics are acceptable, which are taboo; what kinds of confrontations are acceptable, which are not; and other behavioral dimensions such as attendance, taking a break, or leaving the session early.

THE NURSE LEADER'S COMMUNICATION WITH THE GROUP

Given all of the previous ways of interpreting group communication, the nurse leader has to be aware that there are at least three levels of group communication reflecting several issues at any moment in time: individual concerns, "stage development" issues, and possibly other group dynamic questions (e.g., membership, decision making). Initially, it is difficult for a leader to decide how to respond to the different levels, even if the nurse is sure of her own perception of what is going on.

Suppose that in an initial group meeting, it becomes obvious that the group is testing your limits as a leader. They seem to be in a dependency state (similar to the stages noted by Bion, Tuckman, and Bennis and Sheppard). One group member is nonverbally hostile to you for the whole session. Finally, she says somewhat sarcastically, "So how can you help us?" You would probably be torn between putting her in her place, defending your role, and also wanting to encourage participation and perhaps modeling good communication skills. Also, if the goal of the group was for the group to learn to solve its own problems, you would eventually want the group to handle this member's hostility in a way that kept her as a group member. (In this instance, a nondefensive "In any way I can" is enough of a reply in an initial session.)

A further complication for the nurse leader is that everything he or she says is responded to not only as communication, but as communication *from the leader*. The role relationship between leader and group has all sorts of nuances, one of which is that the group responds differently to the leader at various moments in time. Another is that the group members respond individually to the leader. It also seems that the group members do not realize that they respond differently to leaders than to other members of the group. It may be denied. Leaders do not necessarily have an accurate perception of how group members feel about them.

Your own personal style will also affect how groups respond to you. Leaders who are warm, supportive, and active seem to bring about positive

changes in group members. Other stylistic characteristics that seem beneficial in facilitating positive changes in group members are being able to accept
direct hostility from group members and liking the individual group members. Nurses can develop their own leadership styles by getting feedback
from peers, supervisors, and clients about how they come across in the spirit
of discovery rather than self-blame or judgment. Also, the material in Chapter 3 may be helpful in discovering more about communication style as it
applies to leadership.

An additional issue to consider in figuring out how leaders communicate
with the group is that different types of communication may be effective at
different stages of the group's development. That is, the group may be able to
respond to direct feedback (either positive or negative) at some points but not
at others. Similarly, while being active in general was noted as being related
to positive changes in group members, there will be times when the group
"needs" the leader to be silent so the group can do its own work.

The hardest part of all of this discussion comes when a student asks:
Well, what do I do when Ms. Peterson gets uppity in the self-help group? In
part, the answer is "It depends." What it depends on is how Ms. Peterson gets
uppity (what she communicates), what others say in response (a focal conflict?), how long the group has been meeting (stage of development), the
communication role Ms. Peterson and others seem to play in this issue, the
leader's style, the leader's skills, the context in which the group meets, and its
goals. Also, the group members may intervene effectively and be more
helpful at one moment than the leader. By knowing that each of these issues
exists conceptually, the group leader will be able to come up with effective
communication strategies for handling Ms. Peterson and helping the group,
as a whole and individually, to develop and do its task.

The Nurse–Leader in the Nursing Context

Along with paying attention to group development and to the benefits of the
group to its members, the nurse should also be aware of the role of the group
leader within the nursing context. Nurses and nursing students can be asked
to lead groups in a wide range of settings. Furthermore, there are several
roles the nurse may play in the group. These include:

1. Process observer—watches and listens, takes notes
2. Junior leader—leading the group along with a more experienced
   leader
3. Co-leader—leading the group as an equal partner with another
   person
4. Leader—in charge of the group; may have a co-leader, junior leader,
   or process observer present

Each of these four roles requires increasingly advanced skills and knowledge. Before undertaking the leadership of a group, the nurse should assess
the type of group, the constraints and supports within the system, and the

degree of skill required by the role the nurse is expected to play. Too often, nurses are requested to lead groups when they should be junior leaders. A second danger is that the nurse is in over his or her head as far as the type of clientele. A third danger is the lack of support from the setting, including adequate supervision and back-up if clients develop problems that the group setting is not conducive to handling.

COMMUNICATING WITH FAMILIES

One of the current trends in health care is to emphasize the role of the client and his or her support system in promoting and maintaining health. The "support system" usually refers to friends, acquaintances, and especially family members who often provide important components of client care. Support system members include the parent who gives a child medicine, the child who spends 2 hours a day with an elderly mother who is recovering from a hip replacement, the daughters who rotate taking care of their elderly father who can no longer live alone, and neighbors who make sure a single person recovering from a hospital stay is "OK" on a daily basis.

As these persons are involved in the care and emotional health of the client, it certainly makes sense for the nurse to include them in the care plan and, subsequently, communication about the client, her or his condition, and what needs to be done to help maintain the client at her or his optimal level of health.

Families have become one focus of psychotherapy called family therapy (see Jones, 1980, and Jacobson & Gurman, 1986, for a review). While the nurse does not have to be an experienced family therapist to communicate with family members, having some appreciation of the complexity of families, some reasons for attempting communication with families, some barriers to effective communication with families, and some guidelines for effective communication with families make good sense for improving the communication skills of the nurse.

As anyone who has ever lived in a family knows, families are complicated. Some important aspects include the personalities of each individual, the needs and roles of each individual (including child, parent, wife, husband, sister, brother, worker, student, friend, and so forth), and systematic patterns of communication and behavior between all members of the family, called "family dynamics." Also, a family's way of communicating and behaving around an illness may reflect concerns and fears that are not in the family's awareness.

Given the complexity of families, why even bother to communicate with families? As one nurse we know put it "When you get them all together, they all talk at once and I can't understand anything anyone says." The reasons for attempting to communicate with the family are fairly simple: First, the family is directly involved in the care and recovery of the client. Second, the interaction between family members and the client affects the emotional and physical health of the client. Third, because families (and their communication patterns) are complicated, assuming that simply telling one family member what to do or what the "problem" is may distort information to the disadvantage of the client. Finally, the nurse can work to improve the quality of communication and feelings between family members as part of a client care plan.

At the same time, there are several barriers that work against the nurse's having effective communication with all relevant family members. First is logistical and time problems. It can be quite difficult to get relevant family members together (or even have them come in one at a time) during normal working hours. Work, school, child care, and other commitments frequently make getting a family together for a meeting about one member difficult except on weekends or holidays, times when many nurses are not working. Getting everyone together and listening to them can be quite time consuming.

A second barrier is what can be called an "individual" orientation to health. Most of our training is focused on the individual and his or her physical condition. We are used to having a client with varying degrees of illness or disability; we are not used to having to handle a family system with varying degrees of strengths and weaknesses. Similarly, families themselves do not tend to think about how they all interact to promote wellness, illness, or recovery from illness. When you begin to talk to them about their role and functioning in the recovery or care of a client, you may have to educate the family as to its own abilities and shortcomings.

A third barrier is the complexity of communication patterns in families. It is hard to know who is the family member who will be most reliable in understanding your concerns and instructions, who needs to be given "special" concern, and which family members are not on good terms at a moment in time. We rarely have enough information about the interaction of family members in most health settings to make more than educated guesses as the the "best" way to approach and include families in the care of the relative.

Given the nature of families, the need to communicate with them, and the barriers that hinder effective communication with families, it is important that the nurse has some guidelines for initial contact and interaction with families. These guidelines, summarized below, should help you in many cases. If you find that the family is not cooperating, that communication is lost or systematically misinterpreted, you should suspect that there are problems in the family's functioning that may need attention, either from you or someone experienced in working with distressed families. Many families rally to help their ill members. The family can be one of the most important curative factors in any illness.

Our guidelines for communicating with family members are:

- Find out who the relevant family members are and make some sort of a record or chart with their names, ages, and relationships to help you keep track of the family structure.
- Find out who the major "contact" person is (this is usually a female). Make sure that this person's role is honored, even if she or he is not doing a good job at it.

- Assess the degree of supportiveness in the family. Find out (either through discussion with the client or other family members) which family member(s) are most supportive of your intervention and which are potential "blocks." You may also want to find out why this is so from discussions with them.
- Attempt to include both the contact person and family members who are supportive of your intervention (they may not be the same) in any critical conversations about the client, his or her care, and decisions to be made regarding care.
- Attempt to meet at least once with family members in a "family conference" about the client. During the conference, pay attention to how the family seems to communicate with you and each other. While you may find that you cannot get your points across to them, a family conference can serve to show you how the family is working and can lead to more trust being developed between you and family members, particularly if you are not defensive and spend time listening to their concerns.
- Be particularly sensitive to family concerns about the client. Do so by listening, using paraphrasing and other skills discussed in the earlier chapters, using their major channels of communication, and providing emotional support for them at this time of distress. It is important to remember that the entire family is in some sort of distress when a member is ill, even though they cannot always admit it themselves.

Families of Home-Based Clients

Most family members caring for persons in the home are adults caring for an older person. Families provide 80% of all care to the elderly. Caregivers to the aged are (in order of frequency), spouses, female children, female children-in-law, sons, and other members. There is usually one person, called the primary caregiver, who takes on most of the responsibility for the care of the family member in the home (Edinberg, 1988).

Caregivers face a range of concerns, including how to handle other responsibilities in their lives (including work, children, running a household) as well as the instrumental tasks of care, emotional support, and coordination of services. The nurse who is communicating with a primary caregiver has to balance concern for the client's compliance to the medical regimen with providing support to the caregiver. The nurse may, occasionally, challenge the family member to be sure appropriate care is given and that the family itself is not subject to undue duress.

Also important to remember is that the family member may be in the position of caregiver for many months or years. One effective ongoing service for caregivers is support groups that can be found in many communities for families of such conditions as Alzheimer's disease. When discussing support groups or other forms of assistance, however, the nurse must be careful to convey the message that seeking support is positive and *not* a sign that the caregiver has failed to handle matters successfully.

Guidelines for discussing matters with family members in the home include:

1. Be sure you both can take the time to have a discussion.
2. Discuss these concerns in a room in which both of you feel comfortable.
3. If you are discussing a procedure or specific instructions for care, encourage questions and the writing of key information by the family member.
4. Convey your appreciation of the important role the family member plays.
5. Be on the lookout for signs that the family member is feeling stress, burden, or burnout. It is important to be accepting of these feelings even while you are working with the family member to find a way to mitigate them.
6. Attempt to include the client in discussions about care and concerns of the family. Too often, an older person may be excluded in part because the family is displacing its anxiety on them.

EXERCISE IN COMMUNICATING WITH CAREGIVERS

The following exercise will help you sort out the caregiver's feelings from the needs of the client.

1. Pair up, one of you will be the nurse, the other will be the family member (daughter or son) caring for an older person recovering from a heart attack.
2. The nurse's role is to talk with the caregiver, find out how he or she is doing, and instruct him or her on three procedures.
   a. Be sure the client is turned every 4 hours to prevent bed sores
   b. Be sure the client is encouraged to go to the bathroom with assistance (explain that the client needs physical support to stand, get to the toilet, get on, get off and be supported walking back)
   c. Be sure the client is encouraged to eat meals to help them recover
3. The client's role is to listen, ask questions, and also have one of the following concerns:
   a. No other concern
   b. Fear that the parent will not recover
   c. Anger that the parent is taking you away from your family
   d. "Burnout;" that is, you are feeling overburdened, losing sleep, and so forth
4. In the course of a 5-minute discussion, the nurse should attempt to address any concerns the caregiver has in an open-ended manner.

> **5.** After 5 minutes, discuss how the nurse did and whether or not the client felt supported. Then, switch roles and do the exercise again.
> **6.** Discuss ways in which nurses can provide support to family members.

CONCLUSION

Communication with groups and families represent both a challenge and an opportunity for the nurse. Being aware of the importance of group and family dynamics, as they affect clients and others around them, gives the nurse insight into how to help clients achieve their optimum level of functioning. Being aware of how to communicate in groups and families also gives the nurse the ability to work with a given group or family unit as opposed to focusing solely on the individual client. Finally, being able to communicate with groups and families by appreciating their values and norms can be the basis for learning how to communicate with persons from other cultures, which is explored in the next chapter.

REFERENCES

Bennis, W. F., & Sheppard, H. A. A theory of group development. *Human Relations,* 1956, *9,* 415–437.

Bion, W. R. *Experiences in groups.* New York: Basic Books, 1961.

Corey, G. *Theory and practice of group counseling.* Monterey, Calif.: Brooks Cole, 1984.

Corey, G. et al. *Group techniques.* Monterey, Calif.: Brooks Cole, 1987.

Edinberg, M. A. *Talking with your aging parents.* Boston: Shambhala Publications, 1988.

George, R. L., & Dustin D. *Group counseling: Theory and practice.* Englewood Cliffs, N. J.: Prentice-Hall, 1988.

Jacobson, N. S., & Gurman, A. S. *Clinical handbook of marital therapy.* New York: Guilford Press, 1986.

Jones, S. L. *Family therapy: A comparison of approaches.* Bowie, Md.: Brady, 1980.

Shaw, M. *Group dynamics* (3rd ed.). New York: McGraw Hill, 1980.

Tuckman, B. W. Developmental sequence in small groups. *Psychological Bulletin,* 1965, *3,* 384–399.

Whitaker, D. S., & Lieberman, M. A. *Psychotherapy through the group process.* Chicago: Aldine Publishing, 1964.

Yalom, I. D. *The theory and practice of group psychotherapy* (3rd ed.). New York: Basic Books, 1985.

	Communication
Section IV	**and Special Topics**

The final section of this book is designed to give nurses an overview of communication patterns that are specific to unique nurse–client contexts.

The first context relates to the diversity of cultures that exist between nurses and clients. Health beliefs and practices in four ethnic groups are highlighted. How culture can affect communication within nurse–client interactions is important; however, nursing assessments looking at clients as total persons *regardless of cultural background* is a necessary element of effective communication as well.

The second special communication topic dealing with the AIDS/HIV client requires sensitivity and understanding on the part of the nurse. Several barriers can hinder effective communication with this group of clients; however, nurses can transcend these barriers by following some specific guidelines.

Communicating with elderly, confused, and terminally-ill clients can present some interesting challenges to nurses. Abused and chemically dependent clients (and coworkers) require independent decision-making on the part of the nurse.

We believe that nurses face many new and exciting experiences as we approach the 1990s. Effective communication skills will play a large role in these new experiences.

Special Topics

BEHAVIORAL OBJECTIVES

By reading this chapter and participating in the exercises, students will be able to:

1. Describe how culture and language affect communication and professionals' attitudes in health care settings
2. Describe general characteristics of health communication affected by Black, Hispanic (Latino), Southeast Asian, and Middle Eastern American cultures
3. Interpret guidelines for communicating about AIDS/HIV infection
4. Identify guidelines for communicating with elderly and confused elderly clients
5. Discuss effective communication techniques that can be used with the terminally ill
6. List and discuss guidelines for communicating with suspected client abuse, chemically dependent clients and coworkers
7. Identify guidelines for communicating about health behavior.

COMMUNICATION WITH CLIENTS OF DIFFERENT CULTURES

In health care settings, nurses are likely to have contact with subcultures, that is, a group of persons within a culture who have an identity of their own but are related to the total culture (Murray & Zentner, 1989). Consider the following case situation:

Debbie Jones, a 19-year-old black, unmarried mother has brought her 3-month-old baby into the outpatient pediatric clinic because the baby has a fever. The nurse is filling out the record and taking the infant's temperature before the baby is seen by the physician. The nurse, who is white and also 19 years old, is finding it difficult to empathize with this client. She says to herself, "Why does this mother appear to love the baby so much? Perhaps the only reason she had it was to get the welfare payments."

Ms. Jones notices the nurse's actions toward her and thinks to herself, "That nurse is treating me like dirt! She doesn't understand how much I wanted to have a baby of my own!"

Members of subcultural groups *can* have initial suspicion and fear of nurses because nurses are viewed as being powerful, one-up, and, if from a different racial group, nonempathic; however, this is *not* always the case. In addition, it *can* be the nurses who view the clients as powerless, one-down, and different. From a congruent standpoint, the nurse should be actively involved in maintaining the client's sense of self-worth. By respecting the individual client's dignity, the nurse can be an important therapeutic agent, even when the client is in dire social, economic, or health circumstances.

Many clients from different subcultures are not able to speak or read English. This can present a major communication barrier for the nurses. Clients find that because they are not able to speak English, they cannot express their needs or their feelings. Nurses are called upon to use their ingenuity if they too do not speak the client's native language. In some situations, nurses rely on interpreters to communicate effectively with clients who cannot speak or understand English. Sometimes the communication interactions are planned around the presence of the interpreter. This again presents problems when talking about pregnancy or other sensitive issues. In some instances, the inability to understand clients who are unable to speak English can be more the result of nurses *expecting not to understand* than really not having the ability to converse. In situations where neither the client nor the nurse understand the other's language there can be a high level of anxiety. Try to imagine how one might feel in a foreign country where no one understood English. Often the anxiety level is so high that the words of the person with whom one is communicating do not make any sense at all. On the other hand, if one is comfortable in the situation, he or she can survive with relatively few words and observing nonverbal behaviors to make one's desires known.

Fong (1985) has devised an assessment tool enabling nurses to develop care plans for clients of diverse ethnic groups. She includes such questions as "Does the patient speak English?"; "Does the patient understand common health terms?"; "Can the patient read?"; and "What ethnic behaviors or style of communication does the patient use?" in her assessment tool. These questions are important in considering how to plan health care for an individual from a strong ethnic background.

The nurse has to be sensitive to differences in cultural perceptions about many areas, including the sick role, the role of family, the roles of men and women, and even the symbolic importance of foods and diet. These and other cultural values become important when considering how to teach clients to comply with a medical regimen. Sensitivity to these is also crucial in developing trust. They can be learned if the nurse is willing to be taught by the clients.

Communicating with Clients from Varying Cultural Groups

Our attitudes, beliefs, values, sense of personal relationships, use of language and view of the world are experienced individually but are also to a large part shaped by our cultural backgrounds. Too often, cultural differences are seen as avoidance or difficulty on the client's part rather than viewed as an integral component of the individual's way of life and health. It is only through appreciating cultural differences and learning how to work in varied cultural frameworks that the nurse can truly be an effective health professional. The following short sections are an introduction to aspects of several cultural groups' behavior that can affect communication in the nursing context. These sections are meant to be a beginning. They should *not* be used to categorize all individuals in a given group, nor should they be used to suggest that somehow "normal" American culture (white Anglo-Saxon) is superior to any others.

We have chosen four general cultural groups for our discussion: Blacks, Hispanic Americans (Latinos), Southeast Asian Americans, and Middle East Americans. Blacks are currently the largest minority group in the United States, the other three groups have recently increased in numbers in various acute and chronic care settings in the United States as their numbers have increased in the general population.

Black Americans. It is important to note in any discussion of minorities that ethnic and minority groups are not *homogeneous*. In general, ethnic minorities, particularly blacks, are disproportionately disadvantaged compared to whites. The disadvantages are pronounced in terms of access to all types of health care (Foster, 1988).

Discrimination and racism in the American health care system is evident in several ways in the black population. For example, blacks in the U.S. live an average of 6.5 years less than whites (Spector, 1985), have a 50% higher infant mortality rate, and demonstrate striking differences in morbidity when compared with whites with increased incidences of illness across virtually every disease category.

The experience of hospitalization for the lower and poverty income level black is often a degrading and humiliating experience. One reason is that many hospitals today are refusing admission to members of minority groups who have no health insurance and/or are unable to pay for health care. A second reason is that the hospital still remains a white middle class institution. The values for the hospital have been established on a white middle class value system that has resulted in ignored cultural differences and subsequent ineffective communication interactions. Given these facts, how do nurses communicate effectively with a black client? First, nurses should understand black American culture. The family and interdependent kinship ties are characteristic of both rural and urban black communities. Health care is viewed as a family condition and the responsibility for health care rests not only with health professionals and client but with the extended family as well. The nurse can solicit other family members as aides in caring for the black patient.

Religion is an important aspect in the life of a black client. One of the most common methods of treating illness is prayer. The laying on of hands has also been described quite frequently (Spector, 1985). Nurses must be sensitive to the client's need to meet with a member of the clergy or hospital chaplain who can be helpful as liaisons between the family members and nurse and other health professionals (Government Document, 1982).

Language experts today agree that African languages were not totally destroyed by slavery; rather, they have been combined into a black dialect or an Africanized version of English. Often nurses do not recognize the distinctiveness of black dialect, which is evident in verbal and nonverbal behaviors (nuances, tones, and gestures). Many verbal expressions in English can be traced directly to words and expressions of African origin. For example, some common words that are African survivals are tote (carry), gorilla, elephant, okra, jazz, and sorcery. Many verbal expressions that are incorrect English are not, however, random errors, but again have their origins in the African language. For example, "He sick today," or "She tell me she doctor" reflects the lack of verbs within African language (Smitherman, 1986). A nurse hearing such language usage should be careful *not* to judge the client's competency by how he or she fails to use grammatically correct English. In the past, many blacks preferred to consult white professionals in the health care field. Today, blacks prefer to see black professionals because of the black professional's understanding of the culture and language (Bernstein & Bernstein, 1985). While it is not recommended that either black or white professionals care for any client based on skin color, thereby fostering racism, this tendency does demonstrate the need for an increased number of black nurses.

Some ways to increase communication between nurses and black clients are:

1. Respect the black client as an individual and treat him or her as you normally treat other people.
2. Use proper titles ("Mr"/"Mrs") unless you are on a first name basis with the client.
3. Do not patronize a black person.
4. Determine the black client's degree of understanding especially with reference to medical and hospital jargon by allowing for feedback during the interactional process, rather than making assumptions of competency based on usage of grammatically correct or incorrect English.
5. Be cautious of stereotyping the behavior of blacks. One result of stereotyping is that the victimized group begins to believe the stereotype as well.

South East Asian Americans. There are about 100 identifiable ethnic groups within the overall classification of South East Asian Americans, each group differing and reflecting a unique set of sociohistorical forces (Chae, 1987). Three major groups represented in the United States are the Vietnamese, the Cambodians, and the Laotians.

The recent influx of South East Asian Americans has presented an interesting challenge to the health care system. Of the more than 700,000 South East refugees who have settled in the United States since 1975, over 500,000 are Vietnamese. Vietnamese immigration came in two waves; the first wave in 1975 tended to be younger, more educated, and urban, while the second wave comprising the majority of Vietnamese were older, less educated, and less familiar with Western thought and institutions.

Although many Vietnamese have lived in the United States and have adjusted to this new culture, traditional values often surface in response to illness. Many of the older Vietnamese were raised as Buddhists. One of the four central truths of Buddhism is that life is suffering. This can mean that some Vietnamese clients deal with pain and suffering differently than most clients; they may accept pain and suffering as a sign of their inability to be righteous rather than symptoms of physical illness. Thus, there may be a tendency to remain silent when in great pain or discomfort. In addition, many Vietnamese find it difficult to discuss problems with any person other than family or close friends, leading to a tendency to talk around sensitive subjects with strangers, including health professionals.

Proper form and appearance are very important in South East Asian cultures. The head, the seat of consciousness, is considered a sacred part of the body. Nurses are cautioned to either ask permission or be discrete when touching the head of any South East Asian client. Some gestures such as patting the head are considered offensive (Calhoun, 1986).

In many South East Asian cultures, the family is the basic social unit, with the well-being of the family being more important than achievements of its individual members. The Vietnamese family includes many relatives (the extended family) as well as the nuclear family. Therefore, when an important decision is to be made concerning one's care, the decision might rest with a relative (father, mother, older sibling, or close friend) rather than the client (Leung, 1987; Vuong, 1987). Nurses need to be sensitive to this issue in deciding how to communicate information, that is, key family members should be involved.

South East Asian cultures are characterized by filial piety, a high regard for parental authority. This respect can carry over to authority figures. Many South East Asian refugees have worked with nurse practitioners in refugee camps before arriving in the United States and perceive the nurse as an authority figure. A physician is perceived as an even higher authority figure (Chae, 1987; Legg, 1987).

While the emphasis here has been in interacting with the South East Asians, other Asian groups (Japanese, Korean, and Chinese) share some cultural similarities such as filial piety and the importance of the family unit. They also have some distinct cultural differences. One predominant behavior is the tendency to avoid looking directly into the eye of a person who is considered superior. This can mistakenly be interpreted that the listener is disinterested in the speaker (Armstrong, 1986).

A second difference is the emphasis likely to be placed on a hierarchical social system with inherent distinctions between high/low, young/old, or superior/subordinate. Because of the perceived status of the nurse, for example, a client may respond "Yes" when the client does not really understand as a way of pleasing a superior.

Middle East Americans. This diverse group of people (predominantly Moslem) have been immigrating to the United States in larger numbers within recent years. Countries of origin for Moslems in the United States include Egypt, Jordan, Iraq, Arab Palestine, Pakistan, Iran, and India. United States cities with large Moslem populations are Detroit (Arab Americans) and Los Angeles (Iranian Americans).

Middle East Americans as a group have acculturated fairly rapidly, "blending" into American society (Lipson & Meleis, 1985). A nurse working with Middle East Americans may experience unexpected cultural differences in communication styles. One example is in the area of proximics. Middle East cultures accept individuals standing very close to each other while communicating, within "breathing distance."

Another cultural difference revolves around issues of privacy. Silence may indicate the wish to be left alone. Similarly, questions about personal behavior may be viewed as an unwarranted intrusion, rather than an accepted part of health care.

Nurses can also have some difficulty in communicating with Middle East American clients about time. Because involvement with people is culturally more significant than specific time of events, interruptions such as visitors may be viewed as much more important than procedures or scheduled appointments. Similarly, "later," which may have a timed point of reference for the nurse, may be interpreted as "whenever" in Middle East cultures.

Another issue that affects communication in health care is that it is culturally awkward for Middle East clients (particularly males) to accept a foreign female nurse as a serious equal or superior. The male doctor/patient relationship, however, is ranked much higher by Middle East clients in hospitals.

There are also several nonverbal cues particular to Middle East cultures a nurse should be able to recognize (Armstrong, 1986):

1. Raising eyebrows with the head shaking sideways means "I can't understand or hear."

2. Moving all the fingers of the right hand and pointing upward while the other person is talking means "wait a minute." This may also be done when a nurse has said something that the Moslem client considers to be wrong.
3. Gesturing to come here is done through motioning with the whole hand. In the United States, the same gesture is done with the index finger, a gesture that is considered offensive in Moslem cultures.
4. "No" is conveyed with the head tossed back and a tongue click.

None of these differences means that health is unimportant or that Middle East Americans cannot accept health care or the role of nurses. Rather, they suggest that the nurse respect differences, taking particular care in communicating with Middle East Americans to ensure that cultural differences do not adversely influence health care.

Hispanic Americans. Hispanic Americans (also called Latinos) include Mexican Americans (Chicanos), Puerto Ricans, Cubans, and immigrants from all the Central American countries. The Hispanic population is projected to number 35 million by the year 2000, making this group the largest minority in America (Poteet, 1986). Sixty percent of the 14.6 million Hispanics currently residing in the United States (excluding Puerto Rico) are Mexican in origin, with the vast majority residing in the southwest region of the U. S.

A large majority of this client population is of low socioeconomic status. Poverty prevents many from becoming acculturated and hence socialized into dominant Anglo societal values and views (Mardiros, 1984). For many Hispanics, there is also a language barrier that can make it difficult for nurses to conduct a health assessment. Finally, historically there have been many Hispanic immigrants who entered the country illegally. Although legislation in the 1980s allowed many illegal immigrants to become legal residents of the United States, there are still significant numbers of Hispanics in the United States who are unable to obtain health care because of a fear of being deported.

The man is the ultimate authority in Hispanic culture, with the woman assuming two roles: one as daughter or wife—a primarily subservient role—and the other as the revered mother who makes all the decisions regarding the children. The family, not unlike South East Asian cultures, has a strong and supportive role, often being very involved and present during illness, both in and out of the hospital.

The strength of family support can be both a blessing and a difficulty for the nurse. For example, consider the situation of an elderly Hispanic male patient with a severe cardiac problem who is being cared for in the post coronary unit. His family is likely to want to surround him with their presence and loving support; however, the patient is likely to become fatigued with so many visitors. In such a situation, the nurse needs to be able to communicate concerns about giving the patient time alone to recover to the family as well as realize that the message may have to be repeated to a large group of relatives who will want to visit and provide support.

Many Hispanic clients are bilingual, and their language patterns can vary to include phrases from both languages. Bilingual clients can easily switch from one language to the other, preventing clear communication or understanding in either language. At the same time, a client may not have fluency or extensive comprehension in English even though he or she has a basic command of vocabulary and grammar. Nurses are cautioned to be wary that Hispanics can have difficulty understanding what is written in consent forms (there is a high rate of adult illiteracy); they will often sign assuming that their wishes will be honored by their physician, which is not always the case (Mardiros, 1984).

There is a wealth of folklore in the Hispanic cultures regarding health care. Hispanic clients may self-medicate using unorthodox drugs or procedures that have been recommended by the "brujo" or "shaman," even though they may have full knowledge of their illness and correct medical procedures from their nurse (Ailinger, 1988).

Rather than discount folk medicine or language patterns of Hispanic clients, the nurse can work well with Hispanic clients if he or she first takes time to learn some of the cultural customs. In addition, it is important to respect the role of the family and the difficulty a person from one culture has understanding culturally different medical procedures in a second language.

In presenting some differences in communicating with clients of three diverse ethnic groups, it becomes obvious that an understanding of the different behaviors and values can facilitate communication. Two important points to remember are: if you talk plainly, you have a much better chance of being understood, and if you listen (hearing and understanding what you hear), you will probably understand the meaning the ethnic client is attempting to convey. Here are some additional helpful hints in dealing with clients from other cultures:

1. Have an open attitude and recognize that people do have cultural differences. Your culture determines *your* view but that view may not be shared by the clients you care for.
2. Build a trusting relationship by using your listening skills and providing feedback as often as possible.
3. Communicate by using basic words and simple sentences if there is a language problem. Use nouns rather than pronouns. Paraphrase words that carry complicated meanings such as "work-up" and avoid metaphors and colloquialisms.
4. Take time to learn a few words in the language of the client as a sign of respect.

5. Take time to learn major cultural symbols, holidays, and aspects of the client's life, both to understand the client better and show respect for the cultural group he or she is from.

AIDS/HIV INFECTED (AIDS) CLIENTS

Acquired immunodeficiency syndrome/human immunodeficiency virus (*AIDS/HIV*) infection has become the most feared and least understood public health concern in the last decade. The AIDS/HIV infection is caused by a virus that also causes milder but serious illnesses called AIDS-Related Complex (ARC). The AIDS virus is transmitted by direct contact through the blood stream, usually through direct sexual contact and/or reuse of needles for injected drugs. It is not transmitted through saliva, casual contact, or usual physical contact. Despite fears to the contrary, being related to an AIDS/HIV infected patient or using the same implements (cups, utensils, bathroom) does not expose others to risk of catching the disease (Flaskerud, 1989).

Most people who are currently infected with the AIDS virus have no symptoms. The only way they may know they have the virus is through blood tests, although the virus may be in the body for extended periods of time (up to 3 years in some published reports) before current testing procedures can detect it. In addition, estimates are that between one fifth and one third of people with the AIDS virus will develop full-blown AIDS, but the condition may take up to 10 years to be manifest. All persons who test positive for the virus should consider themselves potential carriers of the disease and take precautions not to infect others (Flaskerud, 1989).

People who have full-blown AIDS/HIV infection are likely to die from the condition, as their autoimmune systems cannot fight diseases. Certain forms of lethal cancer seem to occur for this group as well. The two groups in which AIDS/HIV infection most frequently appears are male homosexuals and IV drug addicts, although other sexual partners of a person infected with AIDS/HIV infection and children conceived by a person with AIDS/HIV infection have a high risk of contracting the disease.

AIDS/HIV infection is particularly difficult to discuss because it is associated with nonsocially unaccepted behavior (homosexuality, drug addiction). The condition is misunderstood, and, because it is difficult to detect immediately, sex partners need to have high trust in each other both in specific sexual behavior and in risking exposure to the disease by choice of other partners. In addition, discussion of preventive measures such as the use of condoms in intercourse becomes difficult because certain religious groups view condoms as violating religious practices and beliefs.

Health professionals, particularly nurses who may have to handle AIDS/HIV infected patients and their personal belongings and bedding, need to have accurate information about AIDS and the opportunity to confront their own values about the behavior that frequently leads to contracting the disease. In addition, caring for AIDS/HIV infected patients, while an increasingly expensive component of the health care system, can be very difficult for the nurse who has to deal with a dramatic deterioration in an individual as well as complicated family dynamics from those around the AIDS/HIV infected patient.

Guidelines for Talking About AIDS/HIV Infection

The following guidelines are recommended for discussing AIDS/HIV infection with a person who has the disease, a person in a high-risk group, or a family member of an AIDS/HIV infected victim.

1. Be sure of your facts.
2. Be aware of your own fears, concerns, and values about high risk category behavior (particularly homosexuality and drug abuse).
3. Appreciate that a client has many questions as well as strong underlying feelings.
4. As in discussions focusing on other potentially lethal conditions, you need to address within yourself that your role as the nurse is not to promote or promise a cure but rather that you are there to assist the person or family member in any way you can.

EXERCISE IN COMMUNICATING ABOUT AIDS/HIV INFECTION

1. Pair up. One member of the pair will be the nurse, the other will be one of the three types of persons listed below.
   a. You are married to someone who is worried about having AIDS/HIV infection.
   b. You are a family member (brother, sister) of an AIDS/HIV infected victim.
   c. You think you might have been exposed to AIDS/HIV infection.
2. Simulate a discussion of the client's concerns for 5 minutes. Then, discuss how you felt as client and nurse. Finally, switch roles and try another of the situations.

The diagnosis of AIDS can mean that a patient will be identified as a likely member of a stigmatized group. This can influence nurses' attitudes and behavior, causing some to avoid physical and social contact with AIDS patients. Some nurses have even exhibited the tendency to blame the infected person for the disease. This leaves patients with AIDS/HIV infection vulnerable to feelings of guilt, self-hatred, and ostracism as well as the commonly recognized feelings of fear, anxiety, depression, and anger that accompany life-threatening illnesses (Flaskerud, 1989).

The challenges in communicating with the AIDS/HIV patients are indeed complex. Because medical science has to date provided the AIDS patient with such limited hopes for a cure, nursing interactions tend to emphasize holistic psychological approaches as well as physical skilled nursing care approaches. (For an excellent summary of physical skilled nursing care management of the AIDS/HIV patient, see Ungvarski, P. Chapter 5, in Flaskerud, 1989).

Two psychological approaches that experienced nurses have used with patients in the hospital setting or clients outside the hospital setting are relaxation and the use of imagery. They are mentioned here because they can be useful and also oftentimes constitute important psychological nursing interventions with the AIDS/HIV infected patient.

Relaxation. Teaching patients basic breathing and relaxation exercises is a learned skill that can become a familiar, integrated part of interventions that nurses apply to their clients. Relaxation is especially helpful to the AIDS/HIV infected patient because it can be used in all stages of the illness, and can benefit AIDS patients by decreasing anxiety and tension, decreasing fatigue, increasing the effect of pain medication, as well as disassociating one's self from the pain.

Benson (1975) believes that four factors are necessary in order for relaxation to occur: a quiet environment, a comfortable position, a mental device such as a word repeated over and over, and a positive attitude. Nurses who are interested in learning and practicing this form of therapy for patients will find an excellent reference in Benson's (1975) *The Relaxation Response* that is the basic work in this area. A more recent book by Dossey et al., (1988) is also an excellent resource.

The Use of Imagery. An additional nursing intervention closely related to relaxation for the AIDS patient is the use of imagery. Imagery can be defined as internal experiences of memories, dreams, fantasies, and visions that are frequently paired to a desired state such as relaxation or freedom from pain. Imagery may involve one, several, or all senses and serves as a bridge for connecting mind, body, and spirit.

Most imagery is visual, although some clients may prefer auditory (e.g., singing a song or listening to music) or kinesthetic (e.g., remembering a good feeling or a comfortable experience) images to help them become relaxed. The major goal of imagery is to relax the busy mind and body in order to focus on particular events (Dossey et al., 1988). It is based on the premise that only one thought is processed in the mind's consciousness at any one time.

AIDS patients can be taught to use imagery to aid in the healing or stabilization of the disease or the disability or negative emotional feeling (e.g., fear or anxiety). For further information on imagery, we refer you to Dossey et al.'s text (1988), Chapter 12.

Communicating with Elderly Clients (65+ Years)

Many elderly clients have some form of sensory impairment that can affect one or all communication channels (Gioiella & Bevil, 1985). By sensory impairment we mean a decline in the functioning of one or more senses, which may be caused by environmental influences as well as aging.

It is helpful for nurses to realize the impact of sensory losses when communicating with the elderly clients. Many elderly persons have decreased visual as well as auditory (45%–50%) acuity (Enelow & Swisher, 1986; Esberger & Hughes, S.T., 1989). Clients who have a major sensory loss in one channel are often forced to compensate with other functioning channels. For example, a client may switch to increased use of the auditory channel because of poor vision. There are clients who have sensory deprivation in the three major channels. Picture the elderly client who wears a hearing aid, has glasses, and in whom the sense of touch is diminished. In addition, he or she might even have dentures, contributing to a gustatory loss.

Some elderly clients tend to deny their illnesses and/or capacity to adapt to age-related conditions. Their illnesses are usually chronic and multiple in nature. Although 80% have at least one chronic condition, when asked to rate their personal health, 85% reported being in good or excellent health (Enelow & Swisher, 1986). Often the nurse can observe the client for signs of depression and anxiety which might be clues as to how the client is feeling physically as well as psychologically.

Elderly clients can also assume the psychological characteristics of ill persons (Chapter 7); they often become more dependent and passive and experience greater anxiety, which results in a lowered feeling of self-worth. In the primary care setting, the nurse may well be the only provider the older client sees. The nurse must be careful not to let his or her own fears of aging or stereotypes of the elderly interfere with the care that is given. Openly sharing concerns such as these with an understanding supervisor or colleague is an effective method of handling some of the discomfort primary care nurses feel with elderly clients.

A discussion of the use of the major channels—auditory, visual, and kinesthetic—in elderly clients and their relationship to communication in nurse interaction follows.

Auditory Loss. Deafness in varying degrees is common in the elderly. Approximately one third of the elderly have minimal to serious hearing loss (Bozian & Clark, 1980). Hearing losses may be caused by a decrease in the overall sensitivity to sound or, even more commonly, to high-pitched sounds. There may be a greater loss in one ear than the other. Disturbances in sleep patterns and fatigue from concentration in order to hear are also characteristic of these clients. Imagine yourself obtaining a health history from a client who has a moderate hearing loss. There are several things you can do:

- If possible, eliminate all background noise and find a quiet area or space to talk.
- Speak slowly in low tones so the client has time to process the information. Do *not* make your voice "sing-song" (Bozian & Clark, 1980).
- Face the client. Remember he or she is using the visual channel, providing his or her eyesight is all right. The client will look at your lips, your facial expression, and your body language.
- Check to see if the person has a hearing aid. If so, the hearing aid can be adjusted to your voice. It is also appropriate to check to see if the aid is switched on and the battery is working.
- Speak in a firm voice. There is a way to raise your voice without yelling. Yelling is condescending to clients and has an adverse effect on the elderly. How often do elderly clients say, "Don't yell at me; I can hear you!" Also, there is an incorrect tendency to generalize the hearing loss to *all* the elderly and thus to speak in a loud voice with all these clients.

Visual Loss. The decline in the ability of the eye's lens to accommodate to lights of different intensity starts in the teen years and can result in serious consequences, with subsequent loss of vision in later years. The elderly client who has no visual problems is rare; it is safe to assume that your client will have some visual loss. With remedial steps and a prescription for glasses, however, clients can usually function effectively. The important thing to remember is that elderly clients usually *do not report* visual problems. They tend to assume poor vision or distorted visual images are part of being old.

If the client has a visual loss, the nurse can communicate by using the auditory channel as the predominant channel (assuming there is minimal to no hearing loss). Because of this the nurse should be aware of what he or she is saying, as well as *how* he or she is saying it: voice inflection, tone, volume. Despite some loss of higher pitched sounds, it is not uncommon for elderly clients to develop keen hearing and be able to hear even whispers at a distance. The feelings underneath verbal expressions are often detected by these clients with amazing clarity, and a direct and honest approach is best when communicating with them.

Some ways nurses can help clients with visual impairment are:

- Made sure lighting is adequate.
- Use large print for reading.
- Use color coding for medications and treatments.
- Watch for depth perception. Paint borders on steps.

Kinesthetic Loss. Older clients often do not respond to changes in temperature, either internally or externally, as younger persons do. Also, the speed of information decoding in the central nervous system may be slow, leading to the "foot-shuffling" seen in some older people. Nurses can:

- Check the water temperature if the client is to have a bath or treatment to make sure it is not too hot.
- Make sure the carpet or tiles on floors are designed so that the client can see his or her feet on the floor, thus giving visual feedback.
- Check the room temperature.

Another related kinesthetic "loss" is the lack of personal touch–contact many older people experience. The use of touch (holding hands, hugging, or an arm around a shoulder) is a powerful therapeutic tool that is difficult to overuse.

Isolation and Loneliness. Isolation and loneliness are two terms used to describe the elderly, although there is some question as to exactly how isolated and lonely most people are.

The nurse who works in primary care settings is likely to encounter many elderly who live alone in neighborhoods with changing ethnic mixes. Because others have moved out or died, the older client may feel particularly isolated during illness, even though family are a local telephone call away.

There is a series of questions the nurse should keep in mind in working with older clients who complain of isolation:

- What is the quality and amount of contact with the family?
- What is the quality and amount of contact with informal social supports (friends, mailmen, bank tellers, etc.)?
- Is the client lonely as opposed to depressed? (That is, is social contact or counseling needed?)
- If the nurse is being identified as a substitute for a child ("You're so much like my daughter or son"), at what point does the identification become a problem in maintaining a therapeutic relationship? Also, at what point does the nurse feel uncomfortable about the relationship?

Communicating with any older client will be most successful if the nurse imagines how he or she would want to be treated in the same situation. Empathy (as opposed to sympathy) and a congruent style (as opposed to blame, placating, superreasonableness, or irrelevance) should form the foundation of the therapeutic nurse–client relationship with older as well as younger clients.

Because the nurse may be the sole provider of services to the older client, the nurses's ability to link the client to appropriate programs and services *after* recovery from illness will influence the future course of the client's health status. Thus, the nurse must be able to communicate effectively and to obtain accurate information from the client, but he or she also must be able to communicate effectively with other services and agencies when taking on the role of advocate for the isolated or lonely client.

Nurses often have to *learn* to accept clients in primary care settings with respect and a positive attitude. It is natural that persons judge others using the value systems of their personal and professional role identities. Thus, novice nurses in primary care systems can fall into the pitfall of letting their subjective feelings determine how they view clients.

- He's old.
- She's poor.
- They are dirty.

The client can also feel put down and say to him- or herself:

- I'm too old.
- I'm too poor.
- I'm too dirty.

The challenge is for the nurse to accept people as they are and not impose "conditions" of acceptance. Nurses do not have to approve of or accept the client's values, nor do they have to change their own values.

Confused Elderly Clients. Most nurses at one time or another come in contact with older persons who are confused. That is, the older client is not oriented to person, place, and/or time, as well as having some impairment of memory, judgment, affect, and cognitive abilities. While it is beyond the scope of this book to explore the causes of confusion (see Edinberg, 1985 and Wolanin & Phillips, 1981 for reviews of this issue), it is important to note that signs of confusion can be due to many causes, including overmedication, alcohol, malnutrition, trauma to the head, psychological reactions to trauma, and depression. This group of causes is frequently referred to as "delirious" reactions, frequently characterized by sudden onset, day–night confusion, and a "clouding" of perception. A second set of causes of confusion are the dementias, the most common of which is senile dementia of the Alzheimer's type.

There is still considerable controversy about the prevalence of dementias. Approximately 5 percent of the elderly have senile dementia of the Alzheimer's type, another 2 to 3 percent have other forms of dementia, and about 7 to 8 percent have a form of delirium. There is also controversy as to their causes and prognosis. We do know that many of the conditions leading to delirium can be reversed with a subsequent return of some, if not all, orientation. Senile dementia of the Alzheimer's type is not reversible or treatable at present. Finally, it is quite difficult to diagnose senile dementia of the Alzheimer's type except as a "rule-out" diagnosis.

Where does this leave us as nurses communicating with the confused older person? First, we are unlikely to be sure of the underlying condition the client has. Second, the client may be frightened, depressed, anxious, and at varying levels of awareness about his or her condition. Third, there may well be difficulty in understanding directions or complicated instructions. Fourth, the client may be at varied levels of alertness (ability to engage in conversation, respond to questions, and so forth). None of these possible circumstances and their underlying conditions means we can give up on the client. None of them means that communication is useless. In fact, we can argue that even more care and concern need to be shown for the client who may be upset, afraid, or anxious about his or her condition.

With these thoughts in mind, the following guidelines are useful in communicating with the confused client (Edinberg, 1988):

- Respond to confusion calmly.
- Respond to confusion with the truth and facts.
- Ask the client to relax and speak slowly.
- Explain instructions clearly and slowly.
- Use all channels in communicating.
- Make questions simple.
- Be concrete rather than abstract.
- Give specific answers to client's questions.
- Do not agree if you do not understand the client.
- Act as if you expect the client to understand.
- While simplifying instruction or questions, avoid baby talk or patronizing.
- Avoid confrontation about confused speech. It may be more effective to explain that you do not understand and have the client repeat what she or he said.
- Do not go along with illusions or confused reasoning. Respond with the facts; if confusion persists, be aware that something else may be going on that warrants psychological or medical intervention. Even if the client refuses to believe you, she or he at least is being treated with the dignity of having access to the realities of his or her situation.

Terminally Ill Clients. Consider the following situation:

An old man is dying. He is sick with cancer and pain. At times he wishes it would end. At other times he cries to himself, wishing he could live long enough without pain to go home from this place, this nursing home.

A woman comes to visit. She sits silently, in tears that cannot be shed now. They have lived for 40 years as husband and wife, sharing the same bed, the birth and growth of children, the birth of grandchildren, and the changes of seasons in their lives together. Yet no words find their way to her lips. She only stays a short while and then gets ready to go back to the emptiness of their home, wondering when it will end and how she will live afterward.

A nurse in the facility, it could be you or me, comes into the room as the woman starts to leave. There is a momentary sense that all is not right, that the pain is felt by all three persons in the room. They all know the man is dying, all are unsure how to put words to their feelings (Edinberg, 1985, p. 57).*

Historically, in this type of situation, most nurses (as well as other professionals) would have turned and left the room, assuming that there was little that could be done or communicated to the dying person and his family member. What few people realized, perhaps, was that by saying nothing and leaving, something was being communicated, a message that implied "There is nothing to do about this, it's better not to talk about it."

Fortunately, thanks to the work done by Kubler-Ross (1969) and others, there has been increasing interest and concern about how to handle communication with the dying and their families. It turns out that much of the hesitancy felt by nurses has been more of a reaction to their own fears or concerns about dying than any reality of the client's condition or desire to discuss his or her feelings about the situation.

The first consideration in communicating with the terminally ill, then, is "How ready am I to talk and listen to others talk about their fears, worries, and concerns about death without becoming defensive?" Even if one feels ready, which can take considerable effort and self-examination, there is still a second consideration: "What is the purpose of communicating with the dying person?" In part, the answer to this question varies, but, underlying practically everything that has been written and learned about the process of death is that the dying person may want to talk about her or his feelings, that empathic communication can lead to a sense of hope (even though there is full knowledge that the client will die), and effective communication can also work towards several important goals: ridding the client of unnecessary fears, decreasing psychological distress, helping family members and the client say their goodbyes or finish "unfinished" business, giving the client as much control over the condition and environment as possible, and providing appropriate reassurance that the care givers really care.

It is important to realize that effective communication can serve to help meet these goals, but does not, in and of itself, guarantee that these goals will be met. The nurse can make sure that she or he is working to meet these goals and does not hinder communication. She or he cannot, however, guarantee that all persons involved in the death process will feel good, complete, or that

---

*Adapted by permission of Prentice-Hall, Englewood Cliffs, N.J.

the process will be easy for anyone involved, however, by being capable of appropriate empathic responses, the nurse will do substantial good in many cases and, as is often the case, the nurse will be the one person with the client and family at a time when they are willing and need to talk about what is going on.

The benefits of communication with the dying and their families are thus multifold. First, there is the benefit of communicating that you care, that you can listen. Second, there is the possibility that, by being available to listen, the client will discuss matters or concerns that can be helped by the process of disclosure to another person. Third, matters may come up that need the nurse's intervention which in turn can benefit the client, such as finding out that the client wants some special food or needs to contact a relative. Finally, communication can help families address painful issues that have the potential for a better resolution than their current state of affairs.

Needless to say, simply being available to communicate and listen to difficult emotional issues does not mean that the nurse has the skills to work with all clients for resolution of painful issues. In fact, one of the most difficult issues facing those working with the dying is that things come up that the nurse feels helpless to change or at least does not have the confidence and skills to handle. Psychologically, it may well be easier to avoid the discussion. At the same time, it is often the nurse who is the only person the client may open up to. It takes a certain degree of emotional strength on the nurse's part to be willing to listen to issues she or he may have no control over or may have little expertise in handling. We strongly advocate taking the risks of listening. Also, there should be strong training, structured emotional support, and continuing education in-service available for nurses who come in contact with terminally ill clients. The benefits to the client and families clearly outweigh the potential harm to the nurse.

One of the more difficult issues relating to communication with the dying client is the issue of knowledge of diagnosis (and prognosis). It is not uncommon for a client not to be told he or she is dying. It is not uncommon for a physician (who has the responsibility for telling a diagnosis) to avoid giving the diagnosis due to family pressure or his or her own discomfort with telling someone that their life is ending. It is not uncommon for a client to deny what has been communicated to him or her. There are several points to be made about this issue. First, the client has the right to know his or her diagnosis and prognosis. Second, at times, there is little utility in telling the client the full story due to the client's emotional condition, although a client's being "not alert" or "confused" is *not* one of them. Third, the family is a consideration in the care of the client. Fourth, the medical practitioner may have difficulty in discussing these matters, including not wanting to give a specific answer to "How long do I have to live?" when specific answers to question such as these do not exist. Fifth, the responsibility of informing the client can be delegated from the physician to another person, including the nurse or clergy member. All of these issues have to be weighed in deciding what and how to communicate the diagnosis to the client and family. Inasmuch as the nurse is congruent and in touch with her or his feelings about death, his or her personal concerns will not become unnecessarily entwined with these other issues in what is a difficult enough situation.

Some discussion questions and/or situations are:

- You have been delegated responsibility to tell a client he or she is dying. How would you feel doing this? What might you say?
- How do you feel discussing death?
- How would you feel as a client not being told or being told you had a terminal illness?
- Why should communication with the dying be "different"?

Most nurses feel they are able to cope with the emotions of dying clients but that often this type of interaction results in uncomfortable feelings. If nurses are able to express their own feelings about death in a small group situation, they are able to undertake the first step in developing mutual trust. If these feelings are accepted by the group, then they are able to express more revealing ones. Nurses who have been able to do this are able to communicate more effectively about death and dying with clients. All the key concepts presented in Chapter 4 are especially important in dealing with terminal clients.

Communicating with Abused Clients

Both child abuse and elder abuse have received growing attention in the popular press as well as in professional literature (Campbell & Humphrey, 1984). Many states have passed legislation that defines abuse (usually direct physical or mental aggressive behavior, including sexual interactions and neglect (frequently related to withholding food, shelter, or assistance needed for basic activities of daily living). Such legislation requires that a health professional who has reason to believe that a parent is abusing a child or an adult is abusing an older adult report the situation to proper authorities for further investigation. In part, such legislation was passed because health care professionals have been reluctant to take the risk of confronting an abusive situation. In addition, the person being abused may surprisingly prefer to remain in a dangerous situation rather than be disloyal to family members (Anderson & Thobaben, 1984).

These circumstances make it quite difficult to talk about abuse with a suspected abuser. Many situations in which you will encounter abuse will be ones in which the abuser can choose to leave the treatment site if you are making them too defensive, such as in an emergency room (Fulmer & Cahill, 1984).

Also, many family systems will effectively resist your attempts to change their behavior. Generally, if you are in a situation where there is evidence of abuse of a child, spouse, or older adult (usually physical evidence consists of unexplainable sores, bruises, accompanied by an inability to explain logically how the bruises got there), you need to inform a superior or appropriate person (some emergency rooms, for example, have trained persons on call to handle potential abuse) immediately about your concern.

At the same time, you need to be able to get information from the client without raising the client's defenses. The purpose of such communication is twofold; first, you want to maintain a relationship with the client; and second, you need to get the story as the client gives it if you are going to report your concerns. You do *not* need to get the abuser to confess to his or her abuse. You also should *not* come across as moralizing or blaming, no matter how enraged you may feel on the inside about such behavior. Abuse of children and the elderly is one of the topics that is likely to bring out frustration and anger in you.

Guidelines follow for talking about suspected abuse of children or older adults.

1. If you suspect that there is abuse, report it to appropriate authorities immediately.
2. If you are in communication with a client and evidence of abuse emerges, remember your goal is to get information from the client or suspected abuser rather than change his or her behavior right there on the spot.
3. Avoid moralizing or blaming the client, even in a subtle fashion (e.g., "Why don't you leave?" or, to a child, "You should live someplace else, it would be safer.").
4. Proceed carefully, appreciating that clients, be they abused or abuser, has many strong feelings and a sense that they should not talk about their "secret" behavior.

EXERCISE IN DISCUSSING SUSPECTED ABUSE

1. Pair up. One partner (*A*) will be a nurse; the other (*B*) will be an older person brought into the emergency room by a spouse. The older person has a suspicious mark on their arm that catches *A*'s eye.
2. *A* is to talk with *B* about the mark for 5 minutes. *B* should decide if the mark has a logical explanation or if it in fact came from the spouse hitting them with an object and let this decision dictate how to answer *A*'s inquiry.
3. When you have finished, discuss in the large group:
   a. What kinds of questions and statements made *B* feel comfortable and trusting?
   b. What kinds of questions and statements from *A* made *B* feel uncomfortable and untrusting?
   c. From *A*'s perspective, what kinds of questions, statements, and communication helped get the story from *B*?

4. Then switch roles, only this time *A*, now the client, will be the parent of a child brought in with a broken arm. Partner *A* should decide if the child (age 3) got the broken arm from falling, or if abuse was involved. This decision should help guide how *A* answers *B*'s inquiry.
5. After the 5-minute interview, discuss the following in the large group:
   a. What kinds of questions and statements made *B* feel comfortable and trusting?
   b. What kinds of questions and statements from *A* made *B* feel uncomfortable and untrusting?
   c. From *A*'s perspective, what kinds of questions, statements, and communication helped get the story from *B*?
   d. What differences are there between child and older adult abuse in terms of your communication as a nurse and how society views the two?
   e. How do you feel about abuse, what kinds of emotional reactions do you have, and how might these (understandable and natural) reactions influence your communication with clients who are suspected or potential abusers?

Communicating with the Chemically Dependent Client

Substance abuse has been called one of the three most pervasive health problems facing our society. Substance abuse includes all forms of addiction to drugs, including alcohol. Estimates of combined figures for alcoholism and drug addiction vary, but at least 10% of the adult population has a substance abuse problem (Smith, 1985; Ames & Kneisl, 1988).

Two key components of substance abuse are *physiological addiction*, the body's physical need for a drug, and *psychological addiction*, having the sense that one needs a drug or drink to handle a problem or to feel good. Both are included in treating substance abuse problems.

Substance abuse is difficult to address because its very nature makes abusers secretive. One major defense used is denial, even when the abuser is confronted about his or her dependency on drugs, including alcohol. Substance abuse affects all members of a family. Substance abuse can be found in young and old alike.

When confronted with evidence of substance abuse, the nurse needs to be able to get more information while maintaining or developing trust with the client. At the same time, the client is likely to be secretive and difficult to reach. The reason for needing more information is that, quite frequently, the first evidence is likely to be modest and can easily be explained away by the client.

Perhaps surprisingly, families will consciously or unconsciously collude to protect the substance abuser from being detected. Many support groups have been developed for families in which there is alcohol or drug abuse, in recognition of the impact addiction has on the entire family.

Guidelines to follow for talking about substance abuse are:

1. If you suspect substance abuse, you have a dual role to develop trust and obtain more information if necessary.
2. You have a secondary nursing role, which is to determine necessary intervention and help the client to accept it.
3. Be honest and discreet.
4. Remember to consider issues of confidentiality when dealing with a substance abuse case.
5. Use skills related to trust and empathy.
6. Examine you own values about abuse as well as any history of substance abuse in your own family to be sure you are not forcing your own judgments or morals on the client.

EXERCISE IN COMMUNICATING ABOUT SUSPECTED SUBSTANCE ABUSE

1. Pair up. One partner will be the nurse, the other a client.
2. Pretend that the nurse is taking an initial health history. (Ask the client some introductory open-ended questions about health and concerns). The client will, in the course of answering the questions, make some statement that is *possibly* related to substance abuse (e.g., "I smoke marijuana sometimes/once" or "I hang out with kids who drink").
3. The client should have decided if this statement is really a sign of substance abuse and act on that decision for the rest of the interview with the nurse.
4. The nurse will question the client to explore this sign, while trying to maintain rapport. At the end of 5 minutes, discuss:
   a. Did the nurse maintain rapport?
   b. Did the nurse manage to get more information about the problem?
   c. Did the client in fact have a substance abuse problem? Then, switch roles and repeat steps 2–4 above.

An organization that is helpful to nurses working in the addiction field is the National Nurses Society on Addictions (NNSA). This organization publishes a newsletter four times a year. It also provides information on treatment and research in addiction, certification for nurses working in the field, and a chemically dependent network. Their address is: 2506 Gross Point Road, Evanston, IL 60201; Telephone (312) 475-7300 (Ames and Kneisl, 1988).

Talking about Substance Abuse with a Coworker

Handling chemical dependency in a colleague is quite different than communicating with clients about chemical dependency for several reasons (Sullivan, 1988):

1. In many cases, you will only have the suspicion that something is wrong. You will be open to self-doubt.
2. You are dealing with an equal, you do not have the implicit authority you have with clients.
3. By dealing with equals, they have more latitude to ignore what you are saying, get angry, or withdraw.
4. There are potential negative consequences for you in attempting to talk with a colleague about dependency. You can be viewed (and talked about) as a gossip, busybody, or know-it-all.
5. You also run the risk of ruining a colleague's reputation if you talk to others about your concern.
6. If the colleague is a supervisor, talking about the issue is even more difficult inasmuch as the supervisor has evaluative responsibilities for your performance.

At the same time, chemical dependency (alcohol or drug use) is important to discuss for several important reasons:

1. Chemical dependency is hazardous to the individual nurse and his or her family, in terms of health, economics, and psychological trauma.
2. A chemically dependent nurse can have impaired judgment that can threaten the well-being of his or her clients.
3. Chemical dependency is a treatable condition.

Too often, others protect the chemically dependent individual by ignoring the signs of dependency, hesitating to talk to others (particularly higher-ups) about it for fear of ruining the coworker's reputation or being incorrect. Nurses who themselves are recovering from chemical dependency, however, have urged other nurses to confront them, to intervene, and *not* to protect them by doing nothing (Sullivan, 1988).

Substance abuse is considered a treatable disease. Many hospitals and other health organizations have employee assistance programs specifically designed to help people overcome chemical dependency. Nurses need to be more assertive with each other to protect their own health as well as the health of the clients they serve.

Guidelines to follow for talking with a coworker about substance abuse and/or chemical dependency are:

1. Be clear about your facts.
2. Be empathic and talk about stress or strains your colleague may feel.
3. Be assertive. Your colleague will in all likelihood deny your allegations, get angry, or refuse to talk about it. You need to be prepared for these reactions and have counter arguments, such as "I know you're angry, but I care enough about you to tell you my concern."
4. If your colleague gets defensive, focus on consequences of their behavior (e.g., "If you continue to be late for work or make these mistakes, your job will suffer" rather than focus on the possible dependency).
5. If you are uncertain how to approach the topic, consult with a superior or Employee Assistance Counselor at your place of work on how to raise the topic with a colleague.

EXERCISE IN COMMUNICATING ABOUT SUSPECTED SUBSTANCE ABUSE WITH A COWORKER

1. Pair up. A will be a nurse concerned about B, another nurse, who has shown signs of substance abuse (e.g., missing work with frequency, unexplained mistakes on the job, some change in behavior pattern).
2. A will take a minute to think about how to raise his or her concerns with partner B and then do so.
3. B will counter with a dismissal of what A is saying.
4. A will attempt to continue the discussion without being angry or defensive, focusing on his or her concern for B as well as consequences of B's continuing behavior pattern.

Then, discuss in the large group how if felt to be partner A, partner B, and create a list of concerns for both the dependent person and the concerned coworker. Also, create a list of ways to help nurses talk about these concerns with potentially chemically dependent nurses. Then switch roles and discuss how the second time is easier than the first time.

Talking About Health Behavior

Health-related behavior, such as diet and (stopping) smoking, is one area in which nurses frequently have responsibility in client care. Along with supportive roles for clients who have specific illnesses such as heart disease, nurses are taking an increased role in educating clients in habit control before there is a specific disease or set of symptoms that suggest the client is at risk for a health problem (Pender & Pender, 1987).

There is, however, quite a difference in communicating with a client who has been referred to you for health education as part of a program and communicating with a client when there is no specific health problem. In the latter case, you have two responsibilities; one, to make contact and ensure follow-through by the client, and two, to provide appropriate guidance and ensure compliance with needed regimen. Some guidelines have been suggested for helping clients quit smoking (McMahon & Maibush), but they are also applicable to other forms of health and habit control as well:

1. Be direct.
2. Tell the client the positive consequences of quitting (or losing weight).
3. Point out the immediate benefits of stopping, such as breath, or, in weight loss, self-satisfaction with the first pound. This is very important for adolescents.
4. Make an effort to seek out those who have particular reasons to develop a readiness to quit (i.e., target special efforts to those in high-risk groups, those with parents who have had health related problems similar to those related to the habit at hand).
5. Support and reinforce constant efforts (you are a potential source of social support and follow-up telephone calls).
6. Avoid "scare tactics," it does no good to point out the disastrous effects of health problems the client might get that are related to the habit at hand.
7. Avoid inducing guilt (e.g., "You'll regret it one day").
8. Avoid negative directives (e.g., "Don't do that").
9. Be brief, convey your information concisely, and remind the client of the benefits of stopping the bad habit.

EXERCISE IN DISCUSSING HEALTH-RELATED HABITS

Form into triads. Decide who is *A*, who is *B*, and who is *C*. *A* will be a client, *B* will be a nurse. *A* will have a health related bad habit (usually smoking or being overweight). *B* will spend a few minutes reviewing the guidelines and have a 5 minute discussion with *A* about the habit, trying to follow the guidelines listed above. *C* will function as a recorder, writing down whatever the nurse (*B*) says. At the end of the 5 minutes, *C* will review what B said and compare it to the guidelines. Discuss in the large group:

1. How the client felt when the nurse followed the guidelines.
2. How the client felt when the nurse did not follow the guidelines.

Then switch roles and do the exercises twice more, so that each member of the triad plays each role.

CONCLUSION

Communication in the nursing context is influenced by the culture and specific conditions with which a client is faced. Major cultural groups, including blacks, Hispanics (latinos), Asians/South East Asians, and Middle Eastern Americans, each have somewhat varying values and group norms that influence how they may interact with health care professionals. In addition, nurses increasingly find themselves communicating with clients about topics such as AIDS/HIV infection, the aging process, confusion, terminal illnesses, family violence, substance abuse, and health behaviors. Being able to successfully handle the complexities of nursing care as well as the divergence of cultures and circumstances facing clients is one of the great challenges facing the nursing profession as it prepares to enter the 21st century.

REFERENCES

AHA/CDC Health Education Project. *Culture-bound and sensory barriers to communication with patients: Strategies and resources for health education.* August, 1982.

Ailinger, R. L. Folk beliefs about high blood pressure in Hispanic immigrants. *Western Journal of Nursing Research,* 1988, *10*(5), 629–636.

Ames, S. E., & Kneisl, C. *Essentials of adult health nursing.* Reading Mass.: Addison-Wesley Publishing Co., 1988.

Anderson, L., & Thobaben, M. Clients in crisis. *Journal of Gerontological Nursing,* 1984, *10*(12), 6–10.

Armstrong, M. Expressions of social conventions and language features in Arabic, German, Japanese, Korean, and their importance in a proficiency oriented classroom, 1986. *ERIC ED 278270.*

Bensen, H. *The relaxation response.* New York: Morrow, 1975.

Bernstein, L. & Bernstein, R. S. *Interviewing: A guide for health professionals* (4th ed.). Norwalk, Conn.: Appleton-Century-Crofts, 1985.

Bozian, M., & Clark, H. Counteracting sensory changes in the aging. *American Journal of Nursing,* 1980, *8*, 473–476.

Calhoun, M. Providing health care to Vietnamese in America: What practitioners need to know. *Home and Healthcare Nurse,* 1986, *4*(5), 14–19, 22.

Campbell, J. E., & Humphrey, J. *Nursing care of victims of family violence.* Reston, Va.: Reston Publishing Co., 1984.

Chae, M. Older Asians. *Journal of Gerontological Nursing,* 1987, *13*(11), 10–17, 46–48.

Dossey, B. M., Keegan, L., Guzetta, C., & Kolkmeier, L. G. *Holistic nursing: A handbook for practice.* Rockville, Md.: Aspen Publishers, 1988.

Edinberg, M. A. *Mental health practice with the elderly.* Englewood Cliffs, N. J.: Prentice-Hall, 1985.

Edinberg, M. A. *Talking with your aging parents.* Boston, Shambhala Publications, 1988.

Enelow, A. J., & Swisher, S. N. *Interviewing and patient care* (3rd ed.). New York: Oxford University Press, 1986.

Esberger, K. K., & Hughes, S. T. *Nursing care of the aged*. Norwalk, Conn.: Appleton & Lange, 1989.

Flaskerud, J. H. *AIDS/HIV infection: A reference guide for nursing professionals*. Philadelphia: W. B. Saunders Co., 1989.

Fong, C. M. Ethnicity and nursing practice. *Topics in Clinical Nursing*, 1985, 7(3), 1–10.

Foster, M. Health visitors' perspectives on working in a multiethnic society. *Health Visitor*, September, 1988, 61(9), 275–278.

Fulmer, T., & Cahill, V. Assessing elder abuse: A study. *Journal of Gerontological Nursing*, 1984, 10(12), 16–20.

Gioiella, A. S., & Bevil, C. W. *Nursing care of the aging client: Promoting healthy adaptation*. Norwalk, Conn.: Appleton-Century-Crofts, 1985.

Kubler-Ross, E. *On death and dying*. New York: Macmillan, 1969.

Legg, V. Perceptions of Vietnamese clients and their health care providers: Health status, needs, quality of care. Research Project, University of Illinois, 1987.

Lipson, J. G., & Meleis, A. I. Culturally appropriate care: The case of immigrants. *Topics in Clinical Nursing*, 1985, 7(3), 48–56.

Liung, B. Cultural considerations in working with Asian parents, *ERIC*, 1987, ED285359.

Mardiros, M. A view toward hospitalization: The Mexican-American experience. *Journal of Advanced Nursing*, 1984, 9(5), 469–478.

McMahon, A., & Maibush, R. M. How to send quit smoking signals. *American Journal of Nursing*, 1988, 88, 1498–1499.

Murray, B., & Zentner, J. *Nursing assessment & health promotion strategies through the life span* (4th ed.). Norwalk, Conn.: Appleton & Lange, 1989.

Pender, N. J., & Pender, A. R. *Health promotion in nursing practice* (2nd ed.). Norwalk, Conn.: Appleton & Lange, 1987.

Poteet, G. W. Ethnic diversity. *Journal of Nursing Administration*, 1986, 16(3), 6.

Smith, K. T. Chemical Dependency (Chapter 21) in W. Geels *Signs and symptoms in nursing: Interpretation and management*. Philadelphia: J. B. Lippincott Co., 1985.

Smitherman, G. *Talkin and Testifyin: The language of black America*. Detroit: Wayne State University Press, 1986.

Spector, R. *Cultural diversity in health and illness* (2nd ed.). Norwalk, Conn.: Appleton-Century-Crofts, 1985.

Sullivan, E. J. Which nurse is likely to become chemically dependent? *American Journal of Nursing*, 1988, 791–794.

Vuong, J. T. Vietnamese cross-cultural adjustment. *ERIC*, 1987, ED286977.

Wolanin, M. O., & Phillips, L. R. F. *Confusion: Prevention and care*. St. Louis: C. V. Mosby, 1981.

Index